Aroma~Care™

Pet Aromatherapy

Francine Milford

Aroma~Care™ Pet Aromatherapy by Francine Milford

Aroma~Care™ is a series of instructional booklets on a variety of uses for essential oils.

FrancineMilford@cs.com
www.ReikiCenterofVenice.com
www.AromaCareBooks.com

ID: 978-0-6151-5171-7

Updated 2018 version

Disclaimer: The information shared in the presentation and contained in this document is for informational educational purposes only, and is not meant to diagnose or be used as a replacement or substitute for professional veterinarian health care or medical advice.

Caution
The techniques, ideas, and suggestions presented in this book are not intended as a substitute for proper medical advice. Any application of the techniques, ideas, and suggestions in this book is at the reader's sole discretion and risk.

Table of Contents

Chapter One
History of Aromatherapy from Ancient to Modern Day Uses

What is Aromatherapy?

The term "Aromatherapy" comes from two words, "Aroma" meaning scent and "Therapy" meaning a treatment for a physical or mental condition. Together, Aromatherapy means treating a physical or mental condition using scent. The scent of essential oils comes from plants that are valued for their therapeutic properties. These scents have been used for more than 5,000 years.

Aromatherapy comes from the premise that many illnesses were found to originate in the mind and that a holistic approach may be necessary for healing both body and mind. When essential oils are properly administered, they produce no harmful side effects and help to mobilize the body's own self-healing equilibrium or psychological well-being to regulate physical imbalances.

Essential oils can affect both the physical body and the spirit. Oils have the ability to directly affect the brain and many psychological and physiological processes. Use of aroma lamps, sprays, and inhalation devices bring the many properties of essential oils to the brain.

Characteristics of Essential Oils

Essential Oils are the *Essence* of the plant. Each plant has its own characteristics, personality, life force and energy (vibration). It is this essence that is the carrier of the plant's energy. This essence is the chemical make-up found in the plant itself. This make- up helps to protect the plant from invaders.

Essential Oils are more than 50 times more powerful in oil than herb form. Oils can be taken from various plant parts such as flowers, leaves, bark, seeds, berries, etc. It takes approximately 4,000 pounds of rose petals to create 1 pound of essential oil-that is one reason that some oils are priced more/less than other.

How Essential Oils work

There are many ways that Essential oils can work on our body. One way is from it being absorbed through the skin. Through the absorption process, essential oils are carrying to the tissues and organ systems of the body and are transported through the fluids of the body such in the lymph and blood systems. Another way essential oils work is through inhalation. When we inhale the aroma, we set into motion our olfactory system which begins with the aroma penetrating our mucus membrane and the hair-like structures of the olfactory nerves called cilia. Cilia relays this information to the brain which then responds to the stimuli by either becoming stimulated, relaxed, happy, sad, etc.

Ancient Uses

6,000 B.C. - Egyptians were distilling their essential oils for use in perfumes and in burial rites, including (embalming the dead).

-Hippocrates, who has been called the 'Father of Medicine,' promoted daily bath and massages using oils.

-It was the Roman Physician, Discorides, that wrote down information for more than 500 medicinal plants.

5,000 B.C. - Chinese medicine was using plants for healing, beauty products, to make fragrant teas and rice (like jasmine), infused oils and incense and more.

1,000 B.C. - In Australia, the Aboriginal people used the Melaleuca species medicinally.

-Native American Indian Shamans in South America was using essential oils to perform their traditional healing work.

-North America, Native American Indians were burning herbs such as sage, cedar and sweetgrass to create a smoke that they used for purification is what is called smudging.

-Aztecs, Incas and Mayans used steam baths, massage and aromatherapy together. They created a Pinewood ointment that they rubbed on the chest for lung ailments, or elsewhere for muscle pain and aches.

- written work of herbalist Galen that set the standard for Europe for over 1,000 years.

-2,000 A.D. The King James Bible references more than 200 oils in the book.

Modern Day Uses

-1700s. Distillation of plants and flowers was very popular and mostly used in Eau de Cologne and perfumes

-1709. Eau de Cologne-a blend of essential oils and 70/90% ethanol was created by Italian Perfumer.

-1187. Lab testing on antibacterial properties of essential oils.

-1920. Maurice Gattefosse-French perfume chemist-becomes known as the 'Father of Aromatherapy.' He records his research on the healing and antibacterial properties of oils in his book *'Gattefosse's Aromatherapie'*. The book was published in 1937 and is still in print today.

-1920s. French chemist Rene'-Maurice Gattefosse' published his findings in his new field of study that he called, 'L'*aromatherapie.*'

1950s. French biochemist, Marguerite Maury, used aromatherapy in the beauty industry.

-1958. Jean Valnet who started using essential oils in his practice and later he published the now classic book, *The Practice of Aromatherapy.*

-1992. King Tut's grave is opened and the world sees how long essential oil aromas last.

-present day. Tidewell Hospice & Pallative Care here in Florida realizes the importance of massage and essential oils and offer these services to their patients. They also offer classes to their staff in the use of aromatherapy. I even attended one of these classes myself as a massage therapist for which they gave me continuing education credits.

-present day. Many cleaning products contain essential oils such as pine, orange and lavender. Many hand, bath and body products contain essential oils.

What to know before you purchase essential oils

Before you make your essential oil purchase, there are a few things that you should know and look out for. Below is a small list that I feel is important consumer information:

Read the label.

Does the label read 'pure', 'genuine,' or 'fragrance'? If so, then you sure know the difference between them. 'Pure' can be a lot of different things to different companies. So don't base your purchase on this word alone. 'Fragrance' does NOT mean that you are purchasing essential oils.

If you are looking for essential oils, then be sure that the label reads, '100% essential oil' on it. Know where your supplier gets their essential oils and what extraction method that they use. Be aware of the companies ethical business standards, quality guarantees, customer support offerings, etc. We will cover more on this topic a little later in this course.

Grade.

Essential oils sometimes come in what is called 'grades.' Lower grades of oils are sometimes sold as higher grades. We will cover this a little more in the next few pages.

Extended.

I   f you read this on the label of essential oils then this means that the bottle contains a carrier oil (usually jojoba) to which some essential oil is added. I am finding this happening where generally the essential oil (such as rose) is so expensive that they add a few drops of it to jojoba in order to sell it the public at an affordable price.

Testing.

The surest way to validate the quality of your essential oil is through a process called Gas Chromatography. This process reports on what chemical constituents are present and in what amounts and is used to verify whether a product reading, '100% pure essential oil' is really just that. We will cover this later on in this course.

Folded.

This is the process of distilling oils several times in order to remove monoterpenes from the oil. This is usually performed on citrus oils.

Rectified or Redistilled.

This is a process of removing a natural component from an essential oil. Some of these natural components include terpene and furocoumarin.

Reconstituted.

This is where an essential oil has a natural or synthetic chemical component added to after they have been through the distillation process.

Intuition and Instinct.

Trust your own instincts and sniff the essential oil. Does the essential oil feel that it has therapeutic value? Is it clear? Does the aroma linger? Our noses know what is real and what is not. Most people with allergies to chemical scents and perfumes, and I include myself in this group, will not have an allergic reaction to pure essential oils. The reason behind that is the fact that pure essential oils do not have the same protein structure as synthetic fragrances and our bodies know the difference between them. Our bodies will accent the protein structure of essential oils but not those of synthetic ones.

Pricing.

One way to perhaps tell if an essential oil is 'real' or not is by its pricing.
Extremely Expensive oils: Rose, jasmine, melissa
Expensive: Frankincense, chamomile, sandalwood
Moderate: Lavender, peppermint, basil
Inexpensive: Eucalyptus, rosemary, orange

Grades of Essential Oil

The first thing that I want to mention here is that there is NO such thing as a "therapeutic grade" essential oil. This is a coined phrase that has come from a pyramid-selling type of company that sells their essential oils. Some companies that are Multi-Level Marketing companies (MLMs) call their essential oils such names as "Therapeutic Grade" or "Pure Therapeutic Grade" or "Certified Pure Therapeutic Grade," etc. This is just their own private labeling brand and does not speak to a national or global standard.

Currently, there are no quality standards or governmental issues to authenticate or judge the quality or performance of essential oils. Hopefully that will change in the future, but for now, any company using these terms are just using them for advertising purposes and as a marketing ploy to lure potential customers in to buy their products. The only for you as the consumer to guarantee the quality of the essential oils that you are purchasing is by using Gas Chromatography and Mass Spectrometry (GC/MS). We will look at this topic a little later on in the course.

For your own information, I have listed below the 'grades' of essential oil that is being promoted by some of these companies. To be sure whether any one company is giving you what you are purchasing, you will have to contact that company directly and ask them questions. To date, there are essentially four grades of essential oils and they are designed by a letter, A through C, and Floral Water.

Grade A essential oils are pure therapeutic quality.
  Pure therapeutic quality
  Usually made from organically grown plants
  Distilled at proper temperatures using steam distillation
Grade B essential oils are food grade.
  Food grade
  May contain carrier oils, chemical additives, fertilizers, pesticides, synthetics, or synthetic extenders.
Grade C oils are perfume grade.
  Perfume grade
  Usually contain solvents

May contain the same type of adulterating chemicals as
listed in Grade B.
Floral Water is a byproduct of the distillation process.
By product of the distillation process

Sources and origins of our Essential Oils

Consumers of essential oils can receive their products from places all over the world. But how do these places affect the quality and constituents of the essential oil? What makes one source of essential oils better than another one?

To help answer these questions, Geoff Lyth from Quinessence Aromatherapy wrote an article titled, "Sources and Origins of our Essential Oils." For his own company, Lyth understands that it takes years of training and testing to learn about the various properties and the organic chemistry of a given species of plant.

Lyth sees that there are few companies that have been in business long enough to gain vital expertise in understanding the many genetic differences in the plant. There is much to learn about the many factors that affect the essential oil of a plant including where it was grown, how it was handled, how it was cultivated and so much more.

But knowing the origin of an essential oil will help you in selecting the right oils to use. An example of this is that if consumers know that the Lavender (Lavandula angustifolia) oil comes from France, then selecting a Lavender essential oil originating in another country may have different properties and as such had different results. This doesn't mean that Lavender coming from a different country is bad; it just means that it will potentially have a different chemistry, odor profile and even a different therapeutic action. Some basic essential oils and their country of origin include the following:

Essential Oils	Latin Names	Origin
Anise Star	Illicium verum	China
Basil*	Ocimum basilicum	Italy
Bay	Laurus nobilis	Morocco
Benzoin	Stryax benzoin	Sumatra
Bergamot	Citrus bergamia	Italy
Birch Sweet*	Betula Alba	USA
Black Pepper**	Piper nigrum	India
Cajeput	Melaleuca cajeputi	Indonesia
Cassia	Cinnamomum cassia	Vietnam
Carnation Absolute	Dianthus caryophyllus	Holland
Carrotseed	Daucus carota	France
Cedarwood*	Cedarus deodora	India
Chamomile German	Matricaria chamonilla	Hungary
Chamomile Roman*	Chameamelum nobile	Hungary
Cinnamon Leaf**	Cinnamomum verum	France
Citronella**	Cymbopogon nardus	Sri Lanka
Clary Sage*	Salvia sclarea	Bulgaria
Clove Bud**	Syzgium aromaticum	India
Coriander	Corriandrum sativum	Russia
Cypress*	Cupressus	France
Eucalyptus	Eucalyptus globulus	China
Fennel Sweet	Foeniculum v. dulce	France
Frankincense*	Boswellia carteri	Ethiopia
Geranium*	Peargoneum graveolens	Egypt
Ginger Root**	Zingiber officinalis	France
Grapefruit Pink	Citrus paradisi	France
Grapefruit White	Citrus racemosa	France
Hyssop*	Hyssopus officinalis	Europe
Jasmine Absolute*	Jasminum grandiflorum	France
Juniper Berry*	Juniperus communis	India
Lavender Bulgarian*	Lavandula angustifolia	Bulgaria

Lavender Croatian*	Lavandula officinalis	Croatia
Lavender French*	Lavandula dentata	France
Lemon**	Citrus limonum	Italy
Lemon Eucalyptus**	Eucalyptus citriodora	Australia
Lemongrass**	Cymbopogon flexuous	India
Lime**	Citrus aurantifolia	Italy
Marjoram*	Thymus mastichina	Spain
Melissa Leaf	Melissa officinalis	Egypt
Mullein*/**	Verbascum thapsus	India
Myrrh*	Commiphora myrrha	Africa
Myrtle	Myrtus communis	France
Neroli	Citrus aurantium	France
Niaouli	Melaleuca viridiflora	New Caledonia
Nutmeg*/**	Myristica fragrans	Indonesia
Orange Sweet**	Citrus sinensis	Brazil
Origanum*/**	Origanum vulgare	France
Palmarosa	Cymbopogon martinii	India
Parsley	Petroselinum sativum	Egypt
Patchouli	Pogostemon cablin	Indonesia
Pennyroyal*/**	Mentha pulegium	France
Peppermint*/**	Menthe arvenisis	Japan
Petitgrain	Petitgrain bigarde	France
Pine (Long Leaf)	Pinus pinaster	USA
Pine (Scotch)	Pinus sylvestris	Hungary
Rose Damask Abs.*	Rosa damascena	Turkey
Rose Geranium*	Pelagonium graveolens	France
Rose Maroc Absolute*	Rosa centifolia	Morocco
Rosemary*	Rosmarinus officinalis	Spain
Rosewood	Aniba rosaeodora	Brazil
Sage*/**	Salvis officinalis	Croatia
Sandalwood Australian	Santalum spicatum	Australia
Sandalwood Mysore	Santalum album	East Indian

Tangerine	Citrus reticulata	Italy
Tea Tree	Melaleuca alternifolia	Australia
Thyme White*	Thymus vulgaris	France
Vanilla	Vanilla planifolia	Brazil
Vetiver	Vetiveria zizaniodes	Java
Violet LeafViola odorata		France
Absolute		
Wintergreen*/**	Gaulgheria procumbens	India
Ylang Ylang	Cananga odorata	France

* Avoid these Aromatherapy Essential Oils during pregnancy
**These Essential Oils can be skin irritants. Avoid if you have sensitive skin.

Aromatherapy Essential Oils are best kept in amber glass bottles to protect them from direct light and heat.
www.AromaCareBooks.com

Aromatherapy and your Pets

Most people who use essential oils on themselves already know the benefits of using Aromatherapy. Unfortunately, some of these people feel that if it is safe and effective for them, it must be safe and effective for their children and pets. Not so.

While dogs have been known to tolerate essential oils very well when used at 1/3 the normal human strength, other pets do not fare so well. In fact, using essential oils on other pets such as cats and birds may actually make them ill.

Cats do not digest the essential oils like humans and dogs do so we must be very careful when even using essential oils in the home, especially if you are spraying the oils on carpets or even into the air. Doing this may be toxic for your cat. If you are in doubt whether the essential oils you are using in your home are making your cat sick, then please visit your pet's veterinarian and ask them for advice.

I have included a cat flea collar recipe in this book but I do not advocate that you use it without consulting your veterinarian first. There is much discussion even among Aromatherapists about what constitutes the right dosage, etc. Do some research on your own; your pets will be that much happier.

One very important safety tip is NEVER to spray or use essential oils in, or around, your pets' eyes or nose. And NEVER have your pet ingest the essential oils. Essential oils are to be used externally only!

Dogs have a much more keen system of smell than humans do so it is very important to make sure you dilute their blends. While it is may not smell like much to you, I promise that it smells pretty potent to them.

Essential oils have been most effective if the treatment of skin problems for dogs. These oils can also discourage fleas from making your dog's nice coat of hair their new home.

Recipes given in this book are for average sized dogs. If your dog is very small, like a Chihuahua, then use a little less of the ingredients. If your pet is much larger, like a Great Dane, then double the recipe. You will need to judge into what size category your dog falls into.

One benefit of using essential oils on your pet is that the natural oils will not harm the sheen of your pet's coat, or dry your pet's skin.

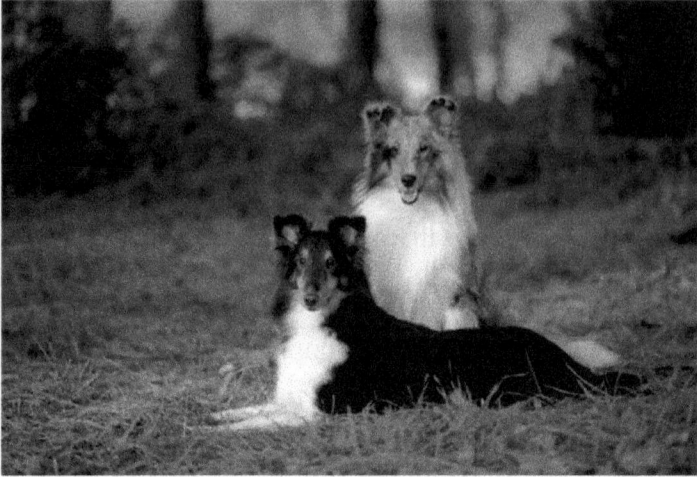

When you pet is suffering from respiratory problems, you can use the same essential oils (in smaller quantities and larger dilutions) on them as you do for yourself. Helpful oils for respiratory problems include eucalyptus, niaouli and tea tree. A nice chest rub recipe will be given in the back of the book.

If you don't like the thought of rubbing essential oils all over your dog's coat, then you can have the options of using alcohol such as brandy or vodka to which you add water.

In fact, when I create a room spray or body spray, I use only spring or distilled water. Remember that essential oils have a shelf life of about 1 month so you will need to discard your blends at that time. That is why it is so important to label all of your blends so that not only will you have an expiration date on the label, but you will also be able to recreate the blend again in the future.

Also remember that oils tends to get stronger, or change, the longer that they 'sit.' A blend that you created yesterday will smell different today and a week from now.

If needed, you can always another drop of essential oil and shake the blend together. Keep in mind that while you may no longer notice a particular essential oil in the blend, your pet sure will.

When first beginning to use essential oils with your pet, start with the smallest amounts of oils and see what your pet's reaction is to them. You can slowly add more oils to your blend but you can't take the oils out of the blend once you put them in-so practice caution.

Read as much information as you can on the subject of using essential oils on your pet. Don't stop at one 'expert.' As the pet owner, it is your responsibility to do the best that you can do to keep you pet healthy and safe, and that means visiting your local library or surfing the Internet for as much information as you can find.

Here is to you and your healthy and happy pet!

Chapter Two
Client Assessment

(For Humans)

The word 'assessment' refers to the process of appraising a client's condition based on both their subjective reporting and your objective findings. This is accomplished in the consultation.

Before and Aromatherapist begins working with a new client, time is set aside for the aromatherapy consultation. This consultation provides the therapists with unique insights into the current needs of the new client. Consultations can be done either in person or on the telephone. When a client comes in person, the client's demeanor can give the Aromatherapist additional information about the health and wellbeing of their client. The Aromatherapist can take a look at the client's skin color and pallor, the client's eyes, the feel of the skin, the way the client walks (fast, slow, limping, crooked, etc.).

A typical consultation will last between 15 minutes to 60 minutes. This session will set up the client-practitioner relationship needed to establish goals and treatment strategies. The Aromatherapist will use this time to identify any underlying issues and prioritize the needs of the systems of the body. The therapist will also look at building a treatment plan and determine the goals for the client, and how long it should take for the client to see any improvement.

The consultation generally begins with the client filling out a detailed client In-take (like the one that follows at the end of this chapter). The In-take should include the following information:

Client Basic Information (name, age, sex, marital status, occupation, address, telephone number, allergies, medications, health history, current health, etc.)

Reason client is seeking aromatherapy

Client's preference for aromatherapy application

Any contraindications

There are three major components to the in-person consultation. These components are:
> **Observation**
> **Interviewing**
> **Evaluation**

Observation

By studying and monitoring your client, Aromatherapists will take into account several factors of their client before deciding on an Aromatherapy blend. Some of the things that the therapists will notice will be the emotional state of their client. Is their client jumpy and easily agitated or are they subdued and lethargic? Are they overweight or underweight? Do they look like they are retaining fluids or have edema? Take a look at their posture. Are they standing straight and tall and move from their hips when they walk, or are they slumped over or look off balance?

Take a look at their muscle tone. Are the muscles taut and is the skin healthy looking or do their muscles sag and their skin look yellowish or pale? Look at your clients' eyes. Do the whites of the eyes look white and clear and do their pupils look moist and shiny or do are the whites of the eyes actually yellowed or bloodshot and are their pupils dry or uneven looking?

Notice your client's voice as they speak. Do they speak with confidence and positivity or is their speech uneven, unsure or even slurred? How is your client communicating their needs and situation to you? Are they hesitating to give up any information or are they like a never ending waterfall of data?

For a successful consultation, it is important for you, the therapists, to take plenty of notes on what you are observing about your client's behavior as listed above. Take note of their expressions and body language.

Do they appear open to sharing their information with you or do they sit back, inattentive and uninvolved in their own treatment plan. Be sure that you implore using active listening techniques which means that not only will you ask open and closed questions, but that you will listen fully to the answers that are given to you.

When you do receive answers from your client, be sure to paraphrase the answers back to you client for verification and or additional information. Be sure to maintain eye contact with your client as it shows that you are involved and care about what they have to say to you.

Also be aware of your non-verbal communication with your client. If you glance at your watch or on the clock on the wall, then you are signaling to your client that you are inpatient. If you glance at your phone that just 'buzzed' a message because you were not professional enough to turn it off, you may give your client the impression that you are not totally in tune with them and their situation, or that you would rather be somewhere else and doing something else. Tapping your pen or nails on the table would also send the message that you are bored with the conversation or impatient with the client.

Be sure that you give your client some feedback to any questions that they are asking you. If you don't know the answer to a particular question, then be honest with them and tell them that. Also be sure to tell them that you will find the information for them and will send it to them, call them with it, or have it ready for them on their next visit. Never judge your client's history or situation as being bad, or good. Try to remain impartial to the issues at hand.

You must also take your client's age and experiences in hand when deciding on what essential oils to blend for them. Always dress and act professionally, maintain eye contact, use proper body language, respect your boundaries and your client's boundaries (which we discuss later in the manual), provide feedback, watch your non-verbal communication, and be observant. One great way to see how you are performed is to go through a mock interview with a friend and video tape the session. When you watch back the session, you will learn a lot about your own strengths and weaknesses.

Interviewing

Therapists will look over the information that client has filled out on the Client In-take form, along with information form observing the client. If the therapist fills that there are areas of information that are incomplete, or that a particular statement needs to be clarified, then the therapist will ask the client open or closed questions.

Closed questions are questions that be easily answered with a 'yes' or 'no' answer or a single word or phrase. Ask closed questions when you want a specific, quick, easy fact and you want to maintain control of the conversation. Open questions are questions that can receive a long answer. Ask open questions when you want your client to think or reflect upon something, give you their feelings or opinions, or when you want them to elaborate.

Open questions usually begin with words such as 'What if' and 'How would you' or 'Why did you' or even 'Tell me how' or 'Describe to me.' The additional information that you gather from the interviewing process will help you in determining how to best help your client. Additional questions may be in regards to any known allergic reactions to plants, nuts, ragweed, flowers, grains, herbs, trees, spices, etc.

At this time, it is also important for me to find out what my client expectations are from me and Aromatherapy in general. What have they tried on their own and what have been their experiences in the past with other therapists and therapies? Does the client has realistic expectations of both my abilities and scope of practice, as well as, what essential oils can and cannot do? If I feel that the client is being unrealistic in the expectations, then this is a time that I use in educating the client in what I, and essential oils, can do for them. If the client agrees with these new realistic expectations, then I will continue with the session. If the client does not agree with these realistic expectations, then I will either close the session or ask some open questions such as, "Why do you believe that this essential oil will perform as you believe?" or "Where have you read the information or data that you believe? This usually helps you in determining the ultimate success you
will have.

Evaluation

Following the consultation, the Aromatherapist will make an assessment of the client's need be going over the information from the client in-take form and observations, and from asking additional questions, etc. The Aromatherapist will then create a blend for the client that will address the client's specific needs.

When finished, the therapist will set out a treatment planning and recommendation for the client. Expectations will be established and how treatment evaluation and review will be taken (weekly, monthly, etc.). Follow-up sessions will be discussed and planned out. Aftercare advice will also be given on follow-up sessions.

The therapist will customize an individual blend for the client, as well as, how the client is to administer the blend (massage, bath, compresses, etc.) The Therapist should give the client a hand out on how often the client is to use the blend and what to do in case of accidental eye contact or ingestion. I like to include contact numbers on this sheet of paper for my own contact information, as well as, poison centers and hospitals.

It is important for the therapist to be contacted if the blend is not working as planned or if something has happened that has made a significant change to the situation, such as being hospitalized or given new medications from your primary healthcare provider, as this may affect you using a given Aromatherapy blend. It is also important to know if the client presents with an allergic reaction to the blend that you have made for them.

A good therapist will document the measurements of the ingredients that they use in a blend for their client. In this way, if they have to replicate the blend again for their client, they will be able to. Be sure to add this document to the client's records along with future notes that speak to the effectiveness of the blend and treatment. You never know if you will use this information in the future for a research project, so be sure that all of your documentation is complete and current.

Client In-take Form

Date_____

Name_____

Address _____

City _____ State _____ Zip Code _____

Telephone(___) _____

Email Address _____

Birthdate _____ Sex _____

Reason for Visit _____

List all of your Medications:_____

How often do you move your bowels every day? _____

How much water do you drink in one day? _____

How much sugar do you consume in one day? _____

How much meat do you consume in one week? _____

How much white flour do you consume? _____

How many dairy products do you eat? _____

Do you feel stressed? Explain_____

Do you have trouble sleeping? _____

Are you pregnant or nursing? _____

Do you have any emotional concerns or needs?_____

Do you have any oils that you like? _____

Do you have any oils that you don't like? _____

The BODY SYSTEM'S QUESTIONNAIRE is below

Client: Circle all numbers in the row that relates to your current issue.

Body Systems	1	2	3	4	5	6	7	8	9	10	11
Abdominal Pain or Discomfort	x	x	x								
Acid indigestion or heartburn	x										
Anxiety, nervousness or tension	x						x	x			
Allergies, Asthma, Hay fever	x	x		X							
Anemia	x					x				x	
Bad breath (Halitosis) or body odor			x		X						

Burning or painful urination					x							
Cold hands and feet						x		x				
Colitis or other bowel irritations		x	x							X		
Constipation or dry stools			x				x					
Dark circles or puffiness under eyes		x			x			x				
Dizziness or light headedness						x		x				
Excess mucous production			x	x								
Fatigue or low energy levels		x	x			x	x	x		x		
Frequent backache					x			x	x			
Frequent cough				x				x		x		
Frequent infections				x				x		x		
Frequent urinary tract infections					x			x				
General weakness or chronic illness	x							x		x		x
Heart Problems						x		x				
High blood pressure					x	x	x	x				
High cholesterol		x			x			x				
Infertility												x
Insomnia		x				x	x					
Intestinal gas, bloating, flatulence	x	x	x									
Joint pain, arthritis or gout					x				x			
Leg cramps or pains					x				x			
Migraine Headaches		x				x	x					x
Muscle aches and pains, stiffness		x	x		x				x	x		
PMS							x					x
Sinus Congestion			x	x						x		
Skin problems		x			x				x	x		x
Stress						x	x					x
Swollen lymph glands (immune system)		x		x						x		
Varicose Veins		x				x			x			
Grand Totals												

	Digestive	Hepatic	Intestinal	Respiratory	Urinary	Circulation	Nervous	Glandular Structural	Immune	Reproductive

<u>For the Professional to fill out</u>
1-Add the total of the circled numbers in each column in the Grand Total above.
2-List the Body Systems from the previous chart that your client circled from 1-10.

(1 will represent the column with the MOST circled x's in it and 10 is the least)
Write down the body system in order from the most x's to the least.
1.
2.
3.
4.
5.
6.
7.
8.
9.
10.
11.

NOTE: Now you have a very good ideal of which of your client's body systems are in most need of help. You have the choice of working on one system at a time, or creating a blend for your client that will take care of several body systems at one time. As each situation and client is unique, you will have to make your best educated guess on how you would like to proceed with your client. If you need help on a particular client, you can drop me an email at <u>FrancineMilford@cs.com</u>.

The Blend Ingredients:
Essential Oils and Number of drops used

_____
_____
_____
_____
_____

Carrier Used _____
Method of Application _____
Length of time to use blend _____
Precautions and Contraindications _____
Additional Recommendations and Information:

_____
_____

Follow-up Date _____

Additional Notes:

Medical History

It is important for you, the therapist, to discover any and all prescription drugs, over the counter medication, and supplements that you client is taking. You will need to know these things so that you do not offer your client an essential oil that can harm them. Below is a list of some popular medications and supplements and their potential negative interactions with essential oils.

Essential oils are fat soluble and can be accessed by the cells in the human body and metabolized by the body. So when there are other drugs present in the body, the active agents of the essential oil may react with that drug in either a positive, negative or neutral way.

Drug Interactions-(Prescription/ Nonprescription)

I encounter the same problems with using essential oils as I do with using herbs in the healing process. Those problems surround people who believe that because essential oils and herbs come from plants and as such are considered 'natural' products, that they can't harm you. This is simply not true. I always treat herbs and essential oils as medicine. In doing so, it helps to remind you to handle and dose with care. You can cause harm if you do not take proper care in preparing blends for your clients.

Some drug interactions may occur during the simple application of just inhaling an essential oil. A highly volatile oil such as Peppermint oil can cause increased lung permeability of nicotine and slow the ability to clear nicotine from the body (Harris, 2008).

Exercise caution when using essential oils in topical application around drug injection side, open cuts or wounds, and around patches (estrogen or nicotine). The wintergreen essential oil has a cortisone-like action because it has a high methyl salicylate, so I would avoid giving wintergreen to clients who are already taking cortisone either internally or topically. In Europe, it is common to see essential oils being given orally, vaginally or rectally. In the United States, we have chosen not to use essential oils orally as this usage must be closely monitored by a medical practitioner or a professional Aromatherapist.

Essential Oil	Avoid Mixing with	Main Body System
Rosemary	Anesthesia, barbituates, May inactivate antibiotics Sedatives (such as barbiturates, benzodiazepines, anesthetics)	Respiratory, Immune
Eucalyptus	Anesthesia, barbituates Sedatives (such as barbiturates, benzodiazepines, anesthetics)	Respiratory
Ravinstara	Anesthesia, barbituates Sedatives (such as barbiturates, benzodiazepines, anesthetics) May inhibit platelet aggregation, May exacerbate blood-thinning action of drugs	Respiratory
Bay laurel	Anesthesia, barbituates Sedatives (such as barbiturates, benzodiazepines, anesthetics)	Respiratory
Wintergreen	Anticoagulant drugs, asthmatics, aspirin allergies. Not for people with ADD/ADHD May cause hemorrhaging in users taking Warfarin (Coumadin, aspirin or Heparin)	Respiratory, Immune, Cardiovascular
Birch	Anticoagulant drugs, asthmatics, aspirin allergies. Not for people with ADD/ADHD May cause hemorrhaging in users taking Warfarin (Coumadin, aspirin or Heparin)	Respiratory, Immune, Cardiovascular
Clove, Clove Bud	Anticoagulant drugs, asthmatics, aspirin allergies (Warfarin, Coumadin, aspirin or Heparin) Antidepressants (MAOI or SSRI drugs, Quinidine, Floxetine and	Respiratory, Immune, Cardiovascular

	Paroxetine, Codeine and Tamoxifen) possible cardiovascular changes prostaglandin inhibitors	
Thyme	Avoid if you have bleeding disorders, major surgery, childbirth, peptic ulcer or hemophilia (Warfarin, Coumadin, aspirin or Heparin) prostaglandin inhibitors May inhibit platelet aggregation, May exacerbate blood-thinning action of drugs	Respiratory, Immune, Cardiovascular
Oregano	(Warfarin, Coumadin, aspirin or Heparin) Avoid if you have bleeding disorders, major surgery, childbirth, peptic ulcer or hemophilia May inhibit platelet aggregation, May exacerbate blood-thinning action of drugs	Respiratory, Immune, Cardiovascular
Cinnamon Leaf	Anticoagulant drugs, asthmatics, aspirin allergies May inhibit platelet aggregation, May exacerbate blood-thinning action of drugs	Respiratory, Immune, Cardiovascular
Allspice Berry	Anticoagulant drugs, asthmatics, aspirin allergies	Respiratory, Immune, Cardiovascular
Pimento Berry	Anticoagulant drugs, asthmatics, aspirin allergies	Respiratory, Immune, Cardiovascular
Niaouli	Increases penicillin and streptomycin	Immune
Lemon	May inactivate antibiotics	Immune
Lemongrass	May inactivate antibiotics	Immune

	Antidepressants such as Bupropion which inhibits CYP2B6 enzyme may influence blood sugar levels	
Lemon Balm	May inactivate antibiotics	Immune
Citrus Eucalyptus Eucalyptus	May inactivate antibiotics Sedatives (such as barbiturates, benzodiazepines, anesthetics)	Immune
Citronellal	May inactivate antibiotics	Immune
Cinnamon Bark	May inactivate antibiotics may influence blood sugar levels May inhibit platelet aggregation, May exacerbate blood-thinning action of drugs	Immune
Orange	May inactivate antibiotics	Immune
Ginger	May inactivate antibiotics	Immune
Melissa	May inactivate antibiotics	Immune
Peppermint	May inactivate antibiotics, Avoid smoking/nicotine calcium channel blocker (felodipine)	Immune, Respiratory, Digestive, cardiovascular
Sage	May inactivate antibiotics	Immune
Spike Lavender	May inactivate antibiotics	Immune
Pennyroyal	May exacerbate glutathione depletion (Acetaminophen)	
Nutmeg	Antidepressants (MAOI or SSRI drugs, Quinidine, Floxetine and Paroxetine, Codeine and Tamoxifen) possible cardiovascular changes	
Holy Basil	Antidepressants (MAOI or SSRI drugs, Quinidine, Floxetine and Paroxetine, Codeine and Tamoxifen)	
Bay (West Indian)	Antidepressants (MAOI or SSRI drugs, Quinidine, Floxetine and Paroxetine, Codeine and	

	Tamoxifen) prostaglandin inhibitors	
Parsley Seed	Antidepressants (MAOI or SSRI drugs, Quinidine, Floxetine and Paroxetine, Codeine and Tamoxifen)	
German Chamomile	Inhibit metabolizing enzymes (CYP2D6) may potentiate the actions of some antidepressants	
Blue Tansy	Inhibit metabolizing enzymes (CYP2D6) may potentiate the actions of some antidepressants	
Yarrow	Inhibit metabolizing enzymes (CYP2D6) may potentiate the actions of some antidepressants	
Balsam Poplar	Inhibit metabolizing enzymes (CYP2D6) may potentiate the actions of some antidepressants	
Geranium	may influence blood sugar levels	
Tumeric	may influence blood sugar levels	
Melissa	may influence blood sugar levels	
Lemon Myrtle	may influence blood sugar levels May inhibit platelet aggregation, May exacerbate blood-thinning action of drugs	
Anise, Star Anise	may influence blood sugar levels Anti-diuretic properties May inhibit platelet aggregation, May exacerbate blood-thinning action of drugs	
Cassia	May influence blood sugar levels May inhibit platelet aggregation, May exacerbate blood-thinning action of drugs	

Fennel	May inhibit platelet aggregation, May exacerbate blood-thinning action of drugs	
Lavandin	May inhibit platelet aggregation, May exacerbate blood-thinning action of drugs	
Marigold	May inhibit platelet aggregation, May exacerbate blood-thinning action of drugs	
Patchouli	May inhibit platelet aggregation, May exacerbate blood-thinning action of drugs	
Tarragon	May inhibit platelet aggregation, May exacerbate blood-thinning action of drugs	
Sedative Oils	May cause too much sleepiness CNS depressants clonazepam (Klonopin), lorazepam (Ativan), phenobarbital (Donnatal), zolpidem (Ambien)	

The Initial Consultation

The first thing that you should do before you begin the initial consultation is to escort your new client to a room that is quiet and private. This is a sensitive matter and should be kept private. Be sure that there is adequate lighting for reading and writing. Be sure that the client feels safe and comfortable. Offer a glass of water if you like. Be sure that you will not be distracted during this time with knocks on the door or with phone calls. This can be very disruptive to the consultation and may send a signal to your new client that you are just not that interested in giving them any personal time.

During the initial consultation, you will have your new client fill out proper documentation in the form of the Client In-take form. You will then write down any of your observations about your client such as their postural analysis, muscle tone, weight, edema, skin sensitivities, allergies, the tone of their voice, their current lifestyle, age, overall health, medication contraindications, and your client's expectations.

The next part of the consultation is finding out what problem they want to deal with first. Which problem made them come to see you in the first place? You will them decide on creating a blend to address your client's specific needs and in what form the application of the blend will take (bath, massage, etc.). Be sure that everything is in writing and that you get your client to sign the form. Date the form. While a client may have many issues when they come to see you, I prefer to work on one issue at a time, if possible. It isn't always possible as several issues can tied in together. But I often let the client choose which issue is the one that they would like most to work on first.

The last part of the consultation session will be me going over the client's expectations for the treatment session to see if it is realistic. If it is not, then I will use this as an opportunity to educate the client on what is, and is not, realistic goal setting.

If a client refuses to fill out the client in-take form, then I will not work with them and I will send them home. I am a professional and as such, I must act accordingly. How can they respect me if I don't even respect my own profession? If they are serious about seeking professional help for their situation, then they will fill out the form. This speaks to my own liability of having a signed consent form from my clients too as we will discuss later on in this manual. We will now take a look at the informed consent form and why this is something important to have signed.

Informed Consent

The informed consent is a client's authorization for professional services based on the information given to them by the therapist. This must be signed by the client after it has been filled out by the therapist. This form will include the therapist's credentials, education and school attended.

Also listed will be any diplomas or certificates or licenses that the therapist has. This will serve as an opportunity for the therapist to lay a foundation of professionalism with the client and to display the therapist's ability to perform the required treatment plan.

Also listed on the informed consent form will be a description of the modalities that will be used, along with the expectations and potential benefits of using said modalities.

In this way, the client will better understand what a potential outcome and result from treatment and what is not.

The form will also contain potential risks and negative side effects of the modalities to be used. In this way, the client will be better able to make a wise and informed decision about their own health care needs. A statement of scope of practice will assure the client that the client does not diagnose a medical condition or prescribe services for medical treatments.

There will also be a *right of refusal* clause in the form where the client has the right to terminate the session for any reason and refuse to be treated by the therapist. This can be done either verbally or written. This works both ways to as you can stop working with a client who make you feel uncomfortable or makes sexual advances towards you. Part of this clause may include information for the client to use in reporting you to the professional board responsible for governing your actions as a therapist.

There should be information on how the client's information and records will be used and stored by you and your facility. You can view HIPAA guidelines to help you create the correct working.

Lastly, there should a paragraph on your office policies and procedures as they deal with client-therapist boundaries, dual relationships, fee schedules and payments, returned checks, canceled payments and missed appointments.

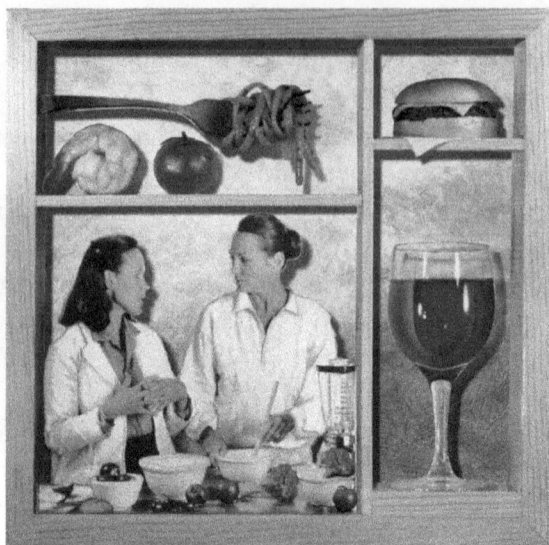

How to Conduct the Consultation (Human)

Have the client fill out a client intake form. If you do not have one, one has been enclosed for you to use with this course.

After the client has filled out the form, look it over and verify the information (to be sure that the client has not made a mistake in filling out the information).

If you have any questions about the information that you are reading, now is the time to verify it with the client.

Ask any additional questions that you feel will help you to set up a plan of action for your client.

Be sure to ask the client what aromas that he/she likes and dislikes.

Begin with the focus of the blend-what goals or actions do you want to help the client achieve first. Having a focus to the blend will help you to narrow down your choices of essential oils that you will use. (A worksheet is included in this manual).

Then write down all of the essential oils that help you to accomplish your goal.

Now that you have your list of essential oils, cross off those that may have contraindications for your client-you can use your reference books to help you here.

Continue to cross essential oils off your list until you have narrowed down your selection to five or seven.

With the five or seven oils that you have, ask the client to sniff each to see which ones the client like, and which one they don't. At the end, be sure to have no more than 5 essential oils left.

Now, decide on which application you will use. With you have the client massage the oils into their bodies? Use compresses? Use a room mist?

After you have decided what application you will use with you client, you can now decide on which carrier oil you will use. Be sure to omit any and all carriers that may be contraindicated for your client. (Like peanut oil for people with nut allergies).

After deciding upon the use and carrier, you will need to decide how many drops of each essential oil you will need to create your blend. A chart is available on the following pages. Be sure to write down how many drops of each essential oil your will use into your notebook so that you can recreate the blend again in the future if you need to.

Blends essential oils first and then add your selected carrier. Shake gently to blend.

Sniff your blend to be sure that you are happy with the result. If you are, then have your client sniff the blend to see their reactions. Don't be surprised if you will have to add an additional drop of oil here or there to please the client's sense of smell.

With your blend completed, create a label with the following information on it:

- Name of the Blend
- Date of the Blend
- Essential oils included in the blend
- ype of carrier
- Directions for use
- How long to use
- Warnings such as 'Keep out of the reach of Children,' etc.
- Protocol to follow in case client accidently gets oil in their eye

Be sure to call your client in a few days to see how the product is working or you can set up a follow up date with your client before they leave you (say in one week). This will give you time to see if your blend is doing the job you were hoping for. If it is not, then you can revisit the situation on the next client visit.

Keep good notes on your client's reaction to the blends that you create. Make it a habit to track your results as this may lead to valuable research findings in the future.

How to Conduct the Assessment (Animal)

In making an assessment of an animal's condition, therapists first determine the cause of any imbalances in the Qi, life force energy. This determination is called the **etiology** of the disease.

It is extremely helpful to the practitioner to find the cause of any discomfort or ailment in order to properly treat it. I often tell my own students to search out the 'root' cause of the illness in order to successfully remove it from the individual, or animal. Sometimes locating this root cause may take more time than you would think. It involves looking at the client, listening to the client, hearing the client, smelling the client, etc. There are many 'clues' that you would look for before you would make a final conclusion as to the treatment plan.

A typical visit to a 'holistic' veterinarian's office may include the following:

- Animal is placed on examining table where its temperature is taken, a physical exam is performed, heart is listened to, bowel sounds are listened to, and the abdomen is palpated to check for any masses. Lab test may be ordered.

- The practitioner would then ask about the dog's behavior and previous history. Asks about the dogs' sleeping patterns, surface preferences to lie on, diet, the animals' environment, stressors, checking tongue, looking at animals body shape, skin and coat. Taking a look at the overall presence of the animal (jittery, lethargic, etc.). Checks the dog's pulse and points along the back that correspond to specific internal organs.

- Check for odors from eyes, nose, ears and mouth.

A typical visit to a holistic practitioner would include:

- Animal is placed on examining table where its temperature is taken, a physical exam is performed, heart is listened to, bowel sounds are listened to, and the abdomen is palpated to check for any masses. Lab test may be ordered.

- The practitioner would then ask about the dog's behavior and previous history. Asks about the dogs' sleeping patterns, surface preferences to lie on, diet, the animals' environment, stressors, checking tongue, looking at animals body shape, skin and coat. Taking a look at the overall presence of the animal (jittery, lethargic, etc.). Checks the dog's pulse and points along the back that correspond to specific internal organs.

- Check for odors from eyes, nose, ears and mouth.

- Decision on which essential oils and application method to use on which point on the body, the length and frequency of the sound therapy session.

If you are not a vet, or have the knowledge of palpating you pet, then I would suggest that you leave this up to a qualified practitioner to perform.

Contraindications

Safety Guidelines and Contraindications of Essential Oils
Because essential oils are popping up on shelves everywhere, the public needs to learn more about how and when to use these oils in a safe environment. Through a lack of knowledge, many people are being hurt by using essential oils. So please, educate yourself on the proper use of essential oils before using them on yourself and others.

General Do's and Don'ts (Human)
- Do not take essential oils internally
- Keep essential oils out of the reach of children and pets
- Keep essential oils out of your eyes and mucous membranes
- Always dilute essential oils in a carrier oil (never apply oils directly to your skin)
- Be sure to use 100% pure essential oils.
- If you are taking Staten medications-avoid hepatoxic oils such as grapefruit.
- Remember that citrus oils are photosensitive. Stay out of sunlight for 12 hours after applying essential oils. Also, avoid tanning beds when using citrus oils.
- Asthma sufferers should avoid steam inhalation as this may irritate and aggravate the mucus membranes. Avoid essential oil of thyme.
- Avoid prolonged use of essential oils. Have 5-6 days on and take 1-2 days off.
- Avoid the essential oil of pine if you have prostate concerns.
- Store essential oils in colored glass containers out of direct sunlight.
- Be sure to use proper dosages for children and pets-do not use adult dosages.
- Use proper ventilation when using essential oils over a long period of time.

- Be sure to perform a Patch Test on yourself before applying essential oils to your entire body, especially if you have sensitive skin.
- Always check with your client about their past reactions to using essential oils.
- Refrigerate carrier oils to prevent them from becoming rancid.
- Old oils are more prone to cause skin reactions. Throw these oils out. Some oils like patchouli and sandalwood get better with age- most do not.
- If you keep a bird in your home, stay away from using essential oils in a diffuser.
- Use caution during pregnancy and while nursing. Safe essential oils include lavender, mandarin and Roman Chamomile.
- If you are allergic to foods like oranges, etc., then you will be potentially allergic to the oils of these products.
- While some oils are effective is used sparingly, they become less effective is you use them too often without a rest.

Consider any cold pressed citrus oil a potential photosensitizer. Steam distilled citrus oils, on the other hand, do not carry this risk. St. John's Wort CO2 and infused oil are also photosensitizers.

Some oils are so dangerous that we have asked you to stay away from using such as: Benzoin, Birch, Bitter Almond, Calamus, Yellow Camphor, Mugwort, Mustard, Rue, Sassafras, Southernwood, Tansy, Thuja, Wintergreen, Horseradish, Wormwood, Verbena, Bay Laurel, Mimosa, Lovage, Tolu Balsam, Ragetes, Peru Balsam, Galbanum Resin, Hyacinth, Oakmoss Concrete, Fig Leaf Absolute.

General Do's and Don'ts (Animal)

Animal Aromatherapy is different from human aromatherapy.

- Avoid use of essential oils with cats, birds, reptiles and fish. This is especially true for using room diffusers or sprays in your environment. Cats and birds to not have the digestive system to metabolize essential oils.
- Just like for humans, do not give essential oils internally to your animals.
- Do not apply undiluted essential oils directly, "neat," to the animal's skin. Always use a carrier oil.
- Just like in humans where you should avoid using essential oils is sensitive areas such as the eyes, nose and mouth-the same holds true for animals. Do not apply essential oils directly to the nose/muzzle, inside ears, near eye or genital areas
- You should use the Patch Test on animals the same that you would do for humans. If irritation occurs, apply a plain carrier oil then wipe off the oil.
- Avoid using essential oils that are photo-toxic on your pets if they will be exposed to sunlight.
- Avoid the essential oils that are on the 'DO NOT USE' list for animals. This chart will found later on in this book.
- Avoid re-applying essential oils to your animals without waiting at least 12 hours between applications.
- Just like for children, keep oils out of reach of animals.

Essential Oil	Avoid
Basil	Avoid during pregnancy, epilepsy, sensitive skin
Bergamot	Photosensitivity
Cassia	Avoid direct sunlight, photosensitivity
Citrus	Avoid direct sunlight
Clary Sage	Avoid during pregnancy (until labor), don't drink alcohol, estrogenic cancers

Clove	Avoid during pregnancy, skin sensitivity
Coriander	Avoid during pregnancy, avoid using too much at one time, kidney problems
Fennel	Avoid during pregnancy, people with seizures
Geranium	Low blood pressure, estrogenic cancers
Ginger	Sensitive skin
Hyssop	Avoid during pregnancy, seizures
Jasmine	Avoid during pregnancy,
Juniper	Kidney problems
Lemon	Photosensitivity
Lemongrass	Avoid during pregnancy, Sensitive skin
Lime	Photosensitivity
Marjoram	Drowsiness, diminish sex drive, decrease sexual function, numb erotic sensations
Melissa	Sensitive skin
Myrtle (lemon)	Avoid during pregnancy,
Myrrh	Avoid during pregnancy,
Oregano	Avoid during pregnancy, skin irritation
Patchouli	Photosensitivity
Peppermint	Avoid during pregnancy, Dilute for high blood pressure
Pine	High blood pressure
Roman Chamomile	Avoid during pregnancy (until labor), drowsiness
Rosemary	Avoid during pregnancy, high blood pressure, epilepsy
Rose	Estrogenic cancers
Sage	Avoid during pregnancy, seizures, high blood pressure
Sandalwood	Kidney problems
Sassafras	Carcinogenic
Tea Tree	Avoid during pregnancy, high blood pressure
Thyme	Avoid during pregnancy, sensitive skin, high blood pressure
Orange (wild)	Avoid direct sunlight
Ylang ylang	Low blood pressure

Chapter Three
Botany

Botany, also called plant biology, is the science of plant life. A botanist is a scientist who studies plant biology. Botanists study some 400,000 species of living organism. Botany actually has its beginning from people who use to identity and cultivate plants for healing call herbalist. Their efforts to identify plants that were medicinal, edible and poisonous were catalogued into collections which were the beginnings of plant taxonomy. On such collections was created by Carl Linnaeus in 1753 and is still in use today.

Modern botany uses new techniques to study plants and analyzes plant chemistry using microscopy and live cell imagine. Botany today looks at the plant chemistry, chromosome number, enzymes, proteins, DNA sequences, etc., to better classify plants.

Botany is concerned with the range and diversity of organisms and their relationships in order to determine evolutionary history. Biological classification is the method by which botanists group organisms into categories such as genera or species and is a form of scientific taxonomy. Carolus Linnaeus grouped species according to shared physical characteristics. This became the beginning of modern taxonomy which now uses DNA sequences as data. The classification order is as follows:

Kingdom
Phylum (or Division)
Class
Order
Family
Genus (plural genera)-First word is capitalized and second is
     lowercase and all is italicized.
Species

To avoid confusion over using a variety of essential oils taken from similar plants, the industry uses Latin names for plant classification. The science of plant classification is called *Taxonony*.

Taxonomy is important because not only will it help you to distinguish one essential oil from another, but also what plant properties you will be getting as each species may offer different therapeutic values.

It is important for you to know not just the common name of the essential oil that you are using, but also its botanical name. In that way, you can be sure that you are using the correct plant and part of the plant to accomplish the result and outcomes that you want to.

Latin names of plants are written as follows:
Families
Genus-(first part of name and first word is capitalized)
Species
Subspecies
Cultivars and varieties
Chemotypes

Families
In biology, the word 'family' represents a taxonomic group that contains one or more genera. Did you know that there are at least three botanical families to the 'chamomile' plant? We have roman, german and moroccan. Each of these plants has different properties and constituents even though they belong to the same botanical family.

To discover more on specific plants, there are several databases that you can go to and look up information on specific plants. One such database is from the University of Florida and can be accessed at: http://edis.ifas.ufl.edu/topic_plant_families.

This database went online in 1995 first as the Florida Agricultural Information Retrieval System (FAIRS) and then three years later changed its name to the Extension Data Information Source (EDIS). It is now considered the single source for all Extension publications and a comprehensive, single-source repository for all peer reviewed publications for free distribution on the web. Funding is provided through the University of Florida Institute of Food and Agricultural Science.

Another free website to go to is from the USDA, Natural Resources Conservation Service at http://www.plants.usda.gov/classification.html. Here you can look up specific information on any number of plants.

In botany, these are the plant families associated with essential oils:

Ericaceae-the 'heather' family.
Betulaceae-the 'birch' family.
Valerianaceae- Now part of the Caprifoliaceae family. 'honeysuckle' family.
Verbenaceae-the 'verbena' family.
Cistaceae-the 'rock rose' family.
Cruciferae-the 'cabbage' gamily.
Liliaceae-the 'lily' family.
Iridaceae-the 'iris' family.
Araceae-the 'inflorescence' family.
Palmae-the 'palm tree' family.
Cyperaceae-'sedges' family.
Moraceae-the 'mulberry' or 'fig' family.
Aristolochiaceae-the 'birthwort' family.
Chenopodiaceae-the 'goosefoot' family.
Ranunculaceae-the 'crowfoot' family.
Euphorbiaceae-the 'spurge' family.
Malvaceae-the 'mallows' family.
Ulmaceae-the 'elm' family.
Podocarpaceae-the 'evergreen' family.
Pinaceae-the 'pine' family.
Taxodiaceae-the 'coniferous' family.
Cupressacaea-the 'cypress' family.

Genus
In biology, the word 'genus' is a taxonomic rank used in classifying living organisms. It is placed below family and above species on the hierarchical scale. The composition of a genus is determined by a taxonomist. The scientific name of a genus is always

capitalized. This name may also be called the 'generic name' or 'generic epithet.'

Species
An example of an essential oil with different species is one of my personal favorite-Eucalyptus essential oil. Some of the names that you may encounter would be the standard, *Eucalyptus globulus,* or it could be *Eucalyptus citriodora* and *Eucalyptus*

Another consideration to keep in mind is that different species also come with different safety guidelines and uses. An example of one such essential oil is Basil. Sweet Basil, *Ocimum basilicum* var. *album* contains less phenolic ethers than its counterpart, Exotic Basil, *Ocimum basilicum* var. *basilicum.*

Cultivars and Varieties
A cultivar is a plant that was selected because of its desirable characteristics (such as resistance to disease, aroma, color, etc.) and maintained by propagation. Examples of this include food crops planted for agricultural, garden plants like roses, camellias and rhododendrons and trees used in forestry that were selected for enhanced quality and yield of timber.

A cultivar name consists of a botanical name (genus, species, infraspecific taxon) followed by a cultivar epithet that is enclosed by single quotes with each of the words within the epithet capitalized. An example of a cultivar name is as follow:
Cryptomeria japonica 'Elegans'

In botany, the word 'variety' is a taxonomic rank below that of a species. It can have an appearance that is distinct from other varieties and it is usually grown geographically separate from other species. Varieties are represented in a three-part infraspecific name. An example would be: The variety *Escobaria vivipara* var. *arizonica* is from Arizona and the *Escobaria vivipara* var. *neo-mexicana* is from New Mexico, but when they meet, they integrate.

Plant Origin and Chemotypes

Where the essential oil comes from can also affect the quality and therapeutic value of the oil. A good example for this is the Sandalwood tree which grows in India but also is being grown now in Australia and other areas of the world. But different minerals exist in the soils of different areas so this will affect the constituents of the oil.

Chemotypes, also known as *chemovars*, is where two plants look identical and cannot be separated out into subspecies, but there are differences between them. These differences exist in the chemical constituents and aroma of the plants. Sometimes the common name of the oil will reflect their chemotype.

Odor and Viscosity of Essential Oils

Essential oils have the properties of odor and viscosity. *Viscosity* refers to the thickness of the essential oil from thin to thick. Thin essential oils tend to evaporate quickly from a blend, thicker oils tend to have odors that last longer and linger on the body for a longer period of time.

The Families of Odor

Family	Scent	Viscosity	Essential Oils
Citrus	Sweet, uplifting	Thin	Bergamot, grapefruit, lemon, lime, orange, tangerine, etc.
Floral	Sweet, euphoric	Thin to Medium	Chamomile, geranium, rose, jasmine, lavender, neroli
Herbaceous	Green, mossy	Thin to Medium	Basil, clary sage, hyssop, marjoram, melissa, rosemary
Woody	Earthy, Smokey	Thin to Medium	Cedarwood, cinnamon, cypress, juniper berry, pine, sandalwood, spruce
Spicy	Pungent	Medium to Thick	Aniseed, black pepper, cardamom, cinnamon, coriander, cumin, ginger, nutmeg
Resinous	Resinous	Thick	Benzoin, elmi, frankincense, myrrh
Camphoaceous	Minty, Earthy	Thin to Medium	Cajeput, eucalyptus, tea tree, peppermint, rosemary, tea
Earthy	Sweet Herbaceous	Medium	Angelica, patchouli, valerian, vetiver

You may blend together essential oils from the same family as listed above.

Chapter Four
Methods of Extraction

There are several ways that essential oils are produced. Below is a list with brief description of each method currently in use today:

Distillation Processes

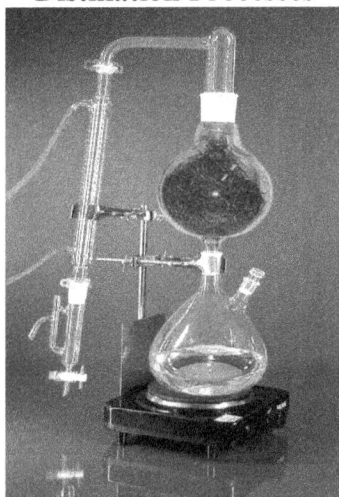

Hydro Distillation
Process of combining the plant material with water kept in the distillation unit. The unit is heated and essential oil is released into steam droplets that rise and are captured and bottled. This method of distillation is a more watered down method of distillation than steam distillation.

Steam Distillation
Here, the plant material is stored in a separate compartment away from the tank of water. As the steam is produced in a boiler it is passed through the plant stored outside the tank. The steam comes from the bottom of the tank. Water vapor comes off the plant and carries the essential oil which is caught, cooled and bottled.

Water or Hydro diffusion

Water diffusion is very similar to steam distillation with one difference; the steam comes from the top onto the botanical material. The condensation of the oil (along with the steam) is hel din place by a grill. In this method, higher oil yields of oils are possible, shorter manufacturing time and less steam is used.

Solvents

Some flowers used to make essential oils contain too little of the volatile oil or are too delicate to undergo expression or the high heat used in steam distillation. For these flowers, a solvent is used to extract the oils. There are many different kinds of solvents that can be used such as petroleum ether, methanol, ethanol or hexane.

Concretes

Extracts using hexane and other hydrophobic solvents. Concretes are a mixture of essential oil, waxes, resins and other plant material.

Absolutes

what is left behind when the alcohol used to extract the essential oil is evaporated. The solvent often used in this process is ethyl alcohol. Plant material is soaked in a solvent (organic chemical like hexane). The mixture of plant material and solvent is called a concrete. Later, the oil is separated from the concrete by using alcohol. This method is often used by perfumeries. The essential oil of Jasmine, Rose and Mimosa is created by this method.

Florasols

A refrigerant used to replace Freon and also used to extract essential oils at below room temperature to keep degradation of the oils.

Carbon Dioxide

This process will extract both the waxes and the essential oil that make up the concrete and then process it with liquid carbon dioxide, which will separate the wax from the essential oil at a low temperature to prevent the decomposition and denaturing of compounds. This is a process often used for making decaffeinate coffee.

Cold Press Extraction (Expression)

This method is the most popular in obtaining citrus oils and is obtained from the rind or peel. This process is also known as scarification. You can accomplish this yourself by placing the plant material between two sheets of glass and placing it out in the hot sun. Droplets of oil with form on the glass-this is the essential oil.

Carbon Dioxide Extraction

This is a relatively new method of extracting essential oils where CO_2 is used to extract the essential oil. This is a very expensive method and is **often used to create essential oils of frankincense and myrrh.**

Hydrosols

Hydrosols are created during the distillation process. When the vapor is released during the distillation process, it mixes with the steam and then separates once cooled. This separation creates the essential oil and the hydrosol. When created from flowers, hydrosols are sometimes called floral water. Unlike oils, hydrosols cannot be synthetically **manufactured in the lab.**

Enfleurage

Enfleurage is the process if placing flowers in a vat of odorless and purified solid fats or oils. The fats/oils absorb the essential oil from the plant material. This method is very time consuming but is much like making an infusion with herbs. (generally 2 weeks).

Hydrosols

Hydrosols are also known as *floral water* and *herbal distillates*. Some see hydrosols as by products from the distillation process or as waste products. So, during the distillation process, there are actually two separate and unique products being created: the essential oil and the hydrosol, or hydrolate.

How this occurs is that during the distillation process, the steam mixes with the plant material and become water and oil. During the cooling process, the water and oil separate creating the essential oil and the hydrolate.

The hydrolate is more than just water; it is water that contains molecules from the plant material and some of the benefits from its mother plant material. Hydrosols are more subtle than essential oils and act more homeopathic. Some popular hydrolates include rose, lavender, and orange.

Since hydrosols still contain some plant material, they must still be handled carefully by either adding a preservative, an alcohol, or kept refrigerated and used quickly. Be sure that the producer of the hydrosol you purchase understands this or you may risk bacterial growth within your product, especially if you are purchasing from someone making oils at their home and may not be well educated in the chemical processes of by-products.

Since there are less chemicals and additives in hydrosols, the essential oil used in these products is much milder and safer. Hydrosols are used primarily in skin care as a body spray, in creams and masks. They can be used in eye inflammations, facial toners, room sprays, astringents (like Witch hazel), cosmetics and toiletries.

Chapter Five
Chemistry

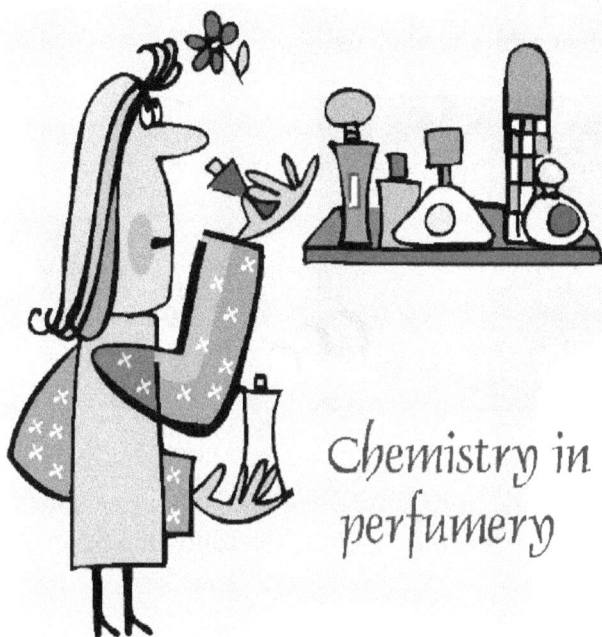

Chemistry in
perfumery

In this chapter, we will cover the following information:
  Atoms and Molecules
  Hydrocarbons
  Monoterpenes
  Diterpenes
  Sesquiterpenes
  Alcohols
  Phenols
  Esters
  Ketones
  Acids
  Aldehydes
  Coumarins
  Oxides

Atoms and Molecules

Atoms are considered the building blocks of live and are the basic components of all substances. Atoms are the smallest unit that exists in a stable form. Each atom consists of a nucleus that is made up of protons and neutrons that orbit the nucleus.

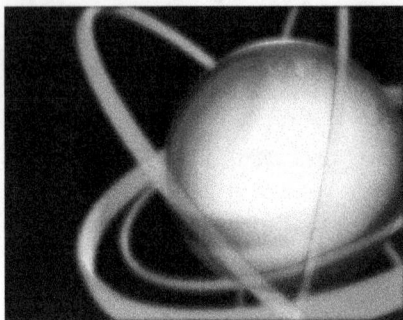

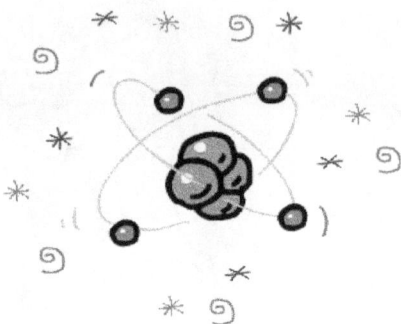

The molecular structures of essential oils contain the elements of life. These elements generally include the following basic elements:
1. carbon (C)
2. hydrogen (H)
3. oxygen (O)

Small amounts of sulphur and nitrogen can also be found at times. When talking about the Chemistry of essential oils, we are talking about the collection of chemical compounds that make up the plant. Below is an example on an essential a-amino acid.

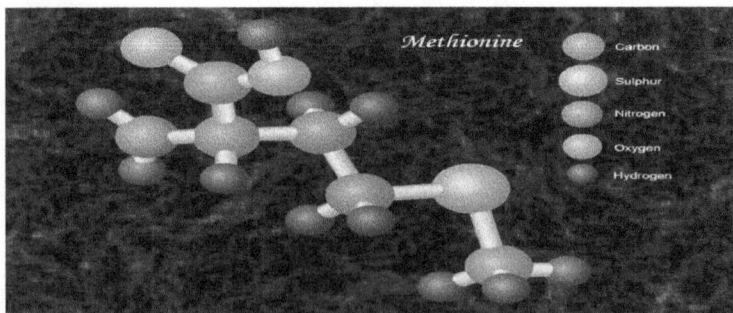

Atoms attract and join with other atoms to stabilize themselves. When atoms come together, they form molecules. Molecules, therefore, are considered compounds because they are made up of more than one element. The type of molecule it becomes is based on the arrangements, number and nature of the atoms that have come together. Almost all molecules that make up essential oils are made from carbon, oxygen and hydrogen. The most often occurring formations are isoprene units which consist of aliphatic chains and aromatic rings.

When we look at organic chemistry, we are looking at carbon based units. Carbon has four chemical bonds that connect it to other carbon atoms where they can form chains and rings. These structures are represented with the letter 'C' to represent carbon, the letter 'O' to represent oxygen, the letter 'H' for hydrogen and 'N' for nitrogen. The bonds between the atoms are presented by a dash.

Examples of common bonds:

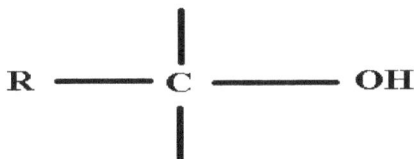

Alcohol

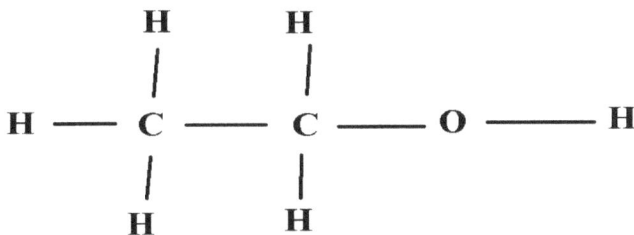

Ethanol

Propanol

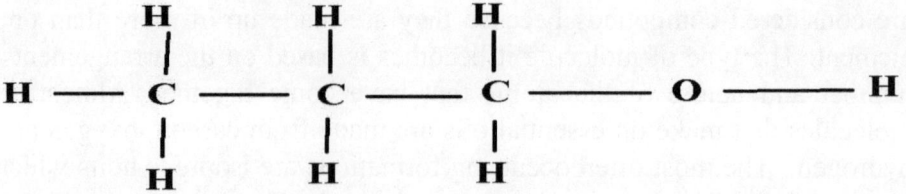

Hydrocarbons

  Aliphatic chains are also known as terpenes and are present in the majority of essential oils. Terpenes are slightly stimulating, may cause skin sensitivity and are antiseptic in nature.

    Monoterpene-(when two isoprene units come together).
    Sesquiterpene-(when three isoprene units come together).
    Diterpene-(when four isoprene units come togeher).

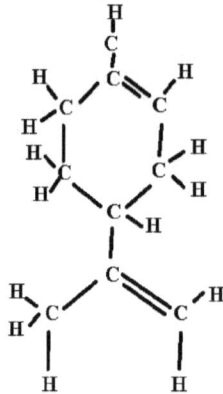

Monoterpene

Terpenes and Essential Oils

Monoterpene-Antibacerial, volatile, highly fragrant, analgesic, and antiseptic. Includes citrus, nutmeg, angelic, pine, fir, spruce and black pepper

Sesquiterpene-Anti-inflammatory, hypotensive and sedative. Essential oils in this: Ginger, patchouli, german chamomile, vetiver, sandalwood, ylang ylang

Diterpene- Horomone balancing, antifungal, antiviral. An essential oil in this group is carrot seed.

The two main groups of compounds

Terpenoids

Phenylpropanoids

Terpenoids-formed along the mevalonate pathway in the plant. This is where the essential oil components are made. These compounds have molecules based on the isoprene unit-5 carbon atoms. These compounds join together to create molecules with 10, 15, or 20 carbon atoms-all multiples of 5. Terpenoids are sometimes called *aliphatic compounds*. These compounds end in "ene" such as lemon (limonene) and juniper (a-terpinene/y-terpinene).

Hemiterpenes=5 carbon atoms
Monoterpenes=10 carbon atoms
Sesquiterpenes=15 carbon atoms
Diterpene=20 carbon atoms
Triterpenes=30 carbon atoms
Tetraterpenese=40 carbon atoms

The aromatic rings are associated with Phenylpropanoids. Rings occur when six or more carbon atoms join together. These rings attract the same types of atoms with similar chemical components. The formation of aromatic rings happens when six carbon atoms join together in a ring, as opposed to a straight or branched chain.

Aromatic rings can attract the same types of atom groups as aliphatic chains to create similar chemical components. The main difference is aromatic rings can form phenols but they cannot form alcohols.

Phenylpropanoids-a smaller group of compounds from the Terpenoids. This group is formed along the shikimate pathway. Their molecules are based on the phenyl ring-6 carbon atoms.

Alcohols-Regarded as non-toxic and uplifting. Recognized for their antiseptic, anti-bacterial and anti-viral properties. Stimulates the immune system, general tonic, and diuretic. The following are components of terpene alcohol:

    Citronellol-eucalyptus, geranium, lemon, rose
    Farnesol-chamomile
    Geraniol-garanium, palmarosa
    Linalol-lavender, rosewood

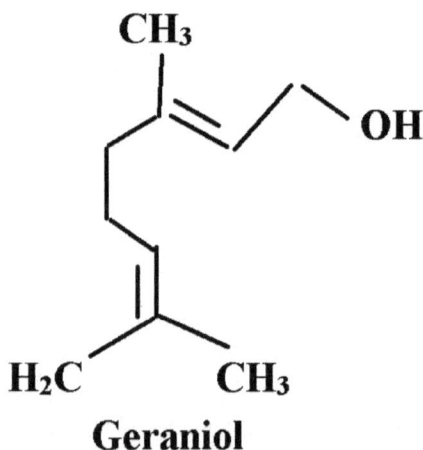

Geraniol

The following are components of sesquiterpene alcohol that are anti-bacterial, anti-inflammatory, anti-mycotic and ulcer-protective:

Bisabolol-chamomile oils

Phenols-Also called, **carbolic acid**, phenols is the 'fragrance' of an
essential oil. Regarded as anti-bacterial, anti-oxidant, antiseptic
and stimulating. Phenols are stimulating and aggressive in their
effects against infection. May irritate the skin or mucus
membranes. Use in small doses for short periods of time.
Phenols whose name ends in 'ol' are part of the alcohol
functional group and is used in pain relief. An example would be
eugenol in clove bud to relieve tooth pain.
Eugenol-cinnamon and clove
Thymol-thyme
Carvacrol-oregano and savory
Methyl eugenol-basil, bay leaf, cinnamon, clove oi,
nutmeg
Methyl chavicol-anise, basil, bay, fennel, tarragon
Safrole-basil, black pepper, cinnamon, nutmeg
Myristicin-dill, parsley
Apiol-dill, fennel, parsley

Naturally occurring phenol

Estradiol	estrogen - hormones
Dopamine	natural neurotransmitters
Adrenaline	natural neurotransmitters
Eugenol	clove essential oil
Methyl salicylate	the major constituent of the essential oil of wintergreen
Salicylic acid	precursor compound to Aspirin
Serotonin	natural neurotransmitters
Thymol	thyme; an antiseptic that is used in mouthwashes
Sesamol	a naturally occuring compound found in sesame seeds

Esters-These are compounds that result from the condensation of an alcohol with an acid and are common in essential oils. Fruit-like odor. Anti-fungal, calming and relaxing. Below is only a sample of some esters and their essential oil connections:

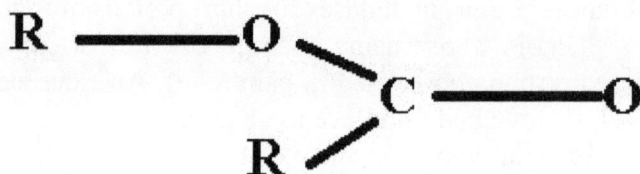

Esters

Ester Name	Odor or occurrence
Allyl hexanoate	pineapple
Benzyl acetate	jasmine
Bornyl acetate	pine
Ethyl cinnamate	cinnamon
Geranyl acetate	geranium
Isopropyl acetate	fruity
Linalyl acetate	bergamot, lavender, sage
Methyl anthranilate	grape, jasmine
Methyl benzoate	fruity, ylang ylang, feijoa
Methyl pentanoate (methyl valerate)	flowery
Methyl phenylacetate	honey
Methyl salicylate (oil of wintergreen)	Modern root beer, wintergreen
Nonyl caprylate	orange
Octyl acetate	fruity-orange

Ketones-Simple compounds that include many sugars (ketoses). Ketons include the industrial solvent acetone which makes it highly prized in industry. Although not highly toxic in general, some essential oils have been flagged (but not documented) to have caused reaction. These essential oils include mugwort, sage, tansy and wormwood. Ketones are used to help with respiratory issues, cell regeneration, tissue formation and mucous.

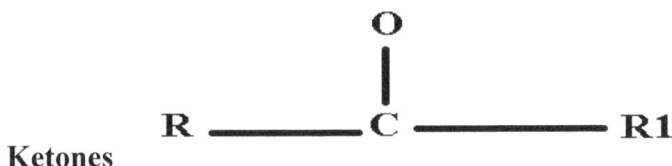

$$R \underline{\quad\quad} \overset{\displaystyle \overset{\textbf{O}}{|}}{\textbf{C}} \underline{\quad\quad} \textbf{R1}$$

Ketones

Ketones
Thujone-Highly toxic irritant to the central nervous system. May relieve respiratory issues and stimulate the immune system when inhaled. Sage and wormwood.
asmone-Jasmine
Fenchone-Fennel
Camphor-Used for respiratory issues (Vick's Vapor Rub)
Carvone-caraway and dill
Menthone-geranium, pennyroyal, peppermint
Methyl nonyl-Also known as 2-Undecanone. Clove and rue oils.

7.) **Acids**-Chemical substances that are characterized by a sour taste, ability to turn blue litmus red, and reacts with bases and certain metals to form salts.
Phosphoric acid-production of phosphate fertilizers, cola drinks
Sulfuric acid-dissolves zinc oxide to product zine
Nitric acid-reacts with ammonia to produce a fertilizer
Carboxylic acids-used with alcohols to produce esters

Acetic acid-vinegar

Carbonic acid-cola drinks, soda, maintains pH equilibrium in the body

Citric acid-preservative in sauces and pickles, citrus fruits, lemon and oranges

Tartaric acid-tamarind and unripened mangoes

Oxalic acid-carambola, rhubarb, spinach and tomatoes

Ascorbic acid-Vitamin C. Found in amla, citrus fruits, guava and lemon

Acetylsalicylic acid-Aspirin. Used to reduce fevers and as an analgesic.

Hydrochloric acid-present in stomach and aids in digestion by breaking down food.

Amino acids-helps to synthesis proteins needed for growth and repair of body tissues.

Fatty acids-required for growth and repair of body tissues

Nucleic acids-helps manufacture DNA and RNA.

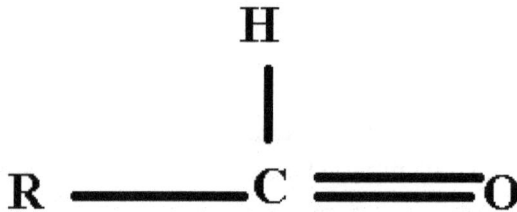

$$R \underline{\hspace{2cm}} C \overset{\displaystyle H}{\underset{}{|}} \equiv\equiv O$$

Aldehydes

8.)**Aldehydes**-Characterized by the group containing carbon, hydrogen and oxygen known as C-H-O. Most sugars are derivatives of aldehydes. Aldehydes are anti-infectious, photosensitive, calming and sedative on the central nervous system (CNS). May be applied topically or via inhalation.

Citral- antiseptic and anti-viral. Melissa oil.

Citronellal-citronella, lavender, lemongrass, lemon, lemon-scented eucalyptus, mandarin, melissa, myrrh.

Benzaldehyde-almonds, apricots, apples, cherry kernels
Cinnamaldehyde-cinnamon bark, powdered cinnamon
Cuminic aldehyde-cumin
Perillaldehyde-perilla

9.) **Coumarins**-'tonka bean.' Analgesic, antiseptic, Anti-arrhythmia, anti-hypertension, anti-HIV, anti-inflammatory, anti-tumor, anti-osteoporosis. Used to treat lymphedema, asthma, autoimmune deficiency, bone loss, inflammation, appetite suppressant, and pain.

First synthesized in 1868, coumarin is used in the pharmaceutical industry as an anticoagulant similar to dicoumarol or the warfarin (Coumadin). Also used as a edema modifier to allow for the body to reabsorb edematous fluids faster. Coumarin is found naturally in the following plants and extracts:

cassia cinnamon (*Cinnamomum cassia*)
deertongue (*Dichanthelium clandestinum*)
Justicia pectoralis extract
mullein (*Verbascum* spp.)
sweet-clover (*Melilotus* ssp.)
sweet grass (*Hierochloe odorata*)
sweet woodruff (*Galium odoratum*)
tonka bean (*Dipteryx odorata*)
vanilla grass (*Anthoxanthum odoratum*)

Coumarin is hepatoxic (toxic to the liver) in rats and moderately toxic to the liver and kidneys in people. The United States Occupational Safety and Health Administration (OSHA) does not classify coumarin as a carcinogen (causing cancer) for humans.

Coumarin is found in some teas, bakery good, strawberries, apricots, cherries, black currants, alcoholic beverages, perfumery, flavors cigarette tobacco and some pipe tobacco (banned in Germany in tobacco use), and in some mulled wine.

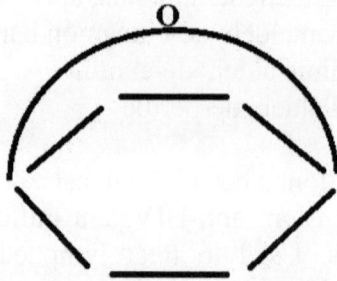

Oxides

10.) Oxides-a chemical compound that contains one oxygen atom and at least one other element. Anesthetic, anti-bacterial, Anti-fungal, and antiseptic.

Cineol (or eucalyptol)- basil, cinnamon, eucalyptus, melissa, ravensara, rosemary
Ascaridol-wormseed oil

Chemical Group	Characteristics	Safety Issues	Essential Oil
Terpenes -or Monoterpenes 'enes'	Stimulates the immune system. Antiseptic. Volatile, Antibacterial, tonic, antiviral, stimulant	Use with carrier oil, possible skin irritant when oil is old, drying to skin	Citrus and Needle oils, pine, cypress, fir, spruce, juniper berry, peppermint, grapefruit, lemon
Sesquiterpenes (strongest odor)	Anti-inflammatory, anti-tumor, liver stimulant, sedative, antiseptic, anti-allergenic, calming		Roots and Woods, Ginger, patchouli, g. chamomile, vetiver, sandalwood, ylang ylang

Monoterpene alcohols	Antimicrobial, sedative, antifungal, antispasmodic, immune supportive	Low toxicity Low irritation	Rose, thyme, geranium, rosewood, citronella peppermint menthol
Sequiterpene alchohols end in "ene"	Anti-inflammatory, antispasmodic, sedative, antiseptic		Sandalwood, nerolina
Diterpene (camphorene)	Horomone balancing, antifungal, antiviral	May be purgative	Carrot seed
Alcohols	Antiviral, uplifting, antibacterial, anti-infectious, immune stimulant, energizing	Non-irritating, great for children and those with sensitivities	Citronella, rose, geranium, eucalyptus, rosewood, palmarosa
Phenols	Antiseptic, antifungal, anti-bacterial, stimulating	May irritate skin and mucous membrane. Hepatoxic	Aniseed, oregano, cinnamon leaf, clove, fennel seed, thyme CT thhymol
Aldehydes End in "al"	Antimicrobial, sedative, hormone balancing	Skin irritant	Melissa, cinnamon, lemongrass, lemon verbena, cinnamon
Ketones End in "one"	Antimicrobial, wound healing	Hepatoxic, Neurotoxic	Camphor, Dill, Spearmint

Esters	Antispasmodic, sedative, adaplogenic, anti-inflammatory	Safe to use	Roman chamomile, cardamom, lavender, clary sage, wintergreen
Lactones (includes coumarins)	Antifungal, antibacterial, mucolytic, expectorant, blood thinner, hypotensive, uplifting, sedative, Coumarins-urinary and coronary dilators	May irritate skin Photosensitivity, Neurotoxic	Inula
Ethers	Antispasmodic, carminative, mucolytic, estrogenic effect, antiviral, decongestant, digestive stimulant	Hepatotoxic	Tarragon, basil, fennel, aniseed, clove, basil, tarragon
Oxides	Expectorant, stimulant, antispasmodic		Eucalyptus, tea tree, spike lavender, rosemary, bay laurel
Sesquiterpinols	Anti-inflammatory, hepatonic, tonic, gland stimulant		Rose, patchouli
Diterpinols	Balances the endocrine system		Clary sage

Chapter Six
The Anatomy and Physiology of the Dog

The following information has been cultivated from many sources including, www.Wikipedea.com from which several images have been put into common use.

The Major Areas of the Dog

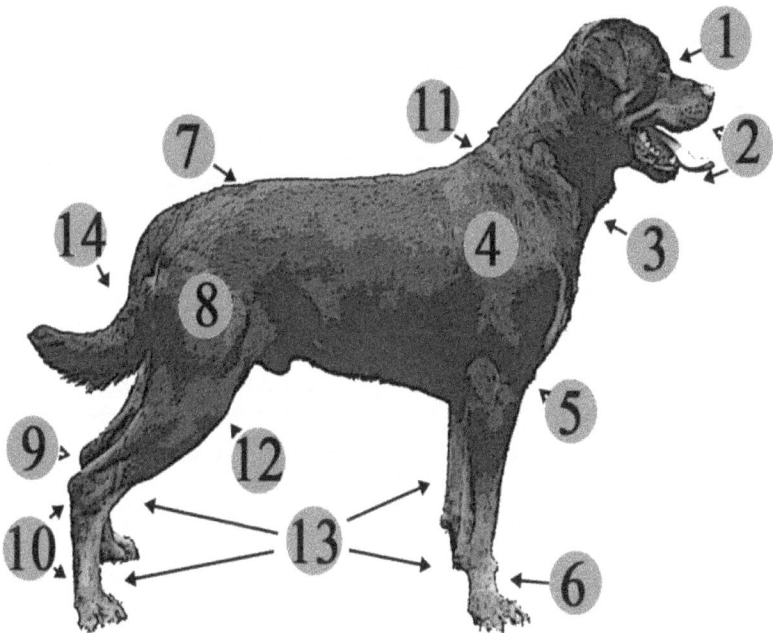

Transferred from de.wikipedia to Commons., based
on Image:Rottweiler.jpg

1. Stop
2. Snout (teeth, tongue)
3. Dewlap (throat, neck skin)
4. Shoulder
5. Elbow
6. Forefeet
7. Highest Point of the Rump
8. Leg (thigh and hip)
9. Hock
10. Hind feet
11. Withers
12. Stifle
13. Paws
14. Tail

Olfaction

Olfaction is how the sense of smell works. It is associated with both the nervous system and the respiratory system. The sense of smell is one of the sensory receptors of our body. Along with the sense of smell we have the following senses: sense of sight (eyes), hearing and balance (ears), and tasting (taste buds). There are other receptors too such as pain receptors that respond to physical damage or injury and thermoreceptors that respond to changes in temperature.

The *olfactory receptors* are located in the small area of epithelial tissue in the upper part of the nasal cavity. These receptors can become very fatigued quickly and after a while they will not be able to sense the odor. This is why we have to 'cleanse our palate' so to speak when we are working with essential oils over a period of time. We can accomplish this by sniffing a container of coffee beans.

Olfactory receptors degenerate over time due to environmental pollutants, smoking and aging. Many older adults suffer from depression with the loss of smell and begin to isolate themselves from other. So, how does the sense of smell work?

With every breath that we take aroma molecules travel a pathway from our nostrils to our brain. This happen thanks in part to a thin layer of sticky mucus that lies at the top of the nose in the epithelium tissue.

Essential oil molecules dissolve in the epithelium tissue and it is then picked up by specialized hair-like receptor cells called *cilia*. From the cilia, the molecules travel to the *olfactory bulb*, the primary organ of smell. This bulb is made up of nervous tissue and contains the only neurons in the body to replace themselves regularly (every 60 days).

In dogs, the olfactory bulb is three times larger than it is in humans which makes them more sensitive to odors and scents.

When we inhale essential oil molecules, a nerve signal in the form of an electrical impulse is sent to the olfactory bulb which process the information and sends it along to the olfactory tract (a bundle of nerve fibers) to the olfactory cortex, and then to the limbic system.

The limbic system is a collection of structures that include the thalamus, the hypothalamus and the amygdale.

The hypothalamus is considered the 'master gland' of the endocrine system and it responsible for regulating several systems of the body such as heart beat, body temperature, hunger, thirst, blood sugar, growth, sleeping, emotions, and more.

Our nose responds in less than 1 second to an odor. Our sense of smell is the only sense that does not need to go through the spinal cord or digestive tract in order to be processed-it can go directly to the brain. The sense of taste is limited to salty, bitter, pungent, astringent, sweet and sour. Our nose can detect approximately 10,000 odors.

About 2 million people in the United States have NO sense of smell. This disorder is called anosmia. A serious head injury can cause anosmia. Most likely this results in damage to the olfactory nerves as they enter the olfactory bulb. It is also possible that damage of the frontal lobes caused by a tumor or surgery can cause anosmia. Elderly people often have a reduced sense of smell.

Researchers Jason Castro from Bates College, Chakra Chennubhotla from the University of Pittsburgh, and Arvind Ramanathan from Oak Ridge National Laboratory published an article in the September 18, 2013 journal **PLOS ONE,** where they identified 10 categories of basic odor qualities. These are as follows:

fragrant
woody/resinous
fruity (non-citrus)
chemical
minty/peppermint
sweet
popcorn
lemon
pungent
decayed

In comparison, the Olfactory System in canines work slightly different than it does in humans. While humans can smell a surface area of 1 in^2 , dogs can cover a surface area of 30 in^2 and where humans only have some 6 million receptors, dogs have approximately 250 million receptors.

The Other Senses

We have already covered the sense of smell previously, but what about the other senses of sight, taste, touch, and hearing? Following is some information on these senses as they relate to your pet.

Hearing

Not only can dogs hear frequencies in the range of 16-40Hz and up to 45-60Hz, but they can also quickly identify in what direction the sound is coming from. In comparison, human hear in the 20-70 Hz and 13-20 kHz range. It takes approximately 18 muscles to raise, lower, tilt, and rotate a dog's ear.

Vision

Dogs have two types of cone photoreceptors which gives them dichromatic vision (they see in only two colors). Dogs can see a part of the range of colors in the visual light spectrum. In comparison, humans have trichomatic vision (they see the three primary colors and the whole light spectrum). For dogs, they are unable to see the range of colors from green to red, making this equivalent to color blindness in human (deutreranopia). When a human sees an object as 'red' in color, the dog will see the same object as being 'yellow' to the dog.

While dogs are less sensitive to differences in grey shades than humans are, they are also 50% less accurate in detecting brightness. But this poor visual acuity does not keep dog's from successfully discriminate between moving objects (which includes identifying their owners in a group of people). They can also see in much dimmer light than humans due to rod cells that 'see' in shades of gray so they need less light to function. Dogs can also see flickering light better than humans but are unable to focus on the shapes of objects which often appear to be blurred to a dog. Some dogs, like Rottweilers, have a genetic predisposition for myopia (nearsightedness).

For more information about dog's vision, etc., please find related articles in the Journal of Veterinary Medicine.

Taste

Dogs have approximately 1,700 taste buds that can taste a variety of different flavors, including that of water (which humans do not have even though they have 9,000 taste buds). Of all of the tastes, dogs dislike bitter tastes the most.

Touch

Above the dog's eyes is a set of whiskers known as vibrissae that are highly specialized sensing organs. These sensing organs are also found in the whiskers below the dog's jar and on their muzzle. The dog uses these whiskers to subtle vibrations, air currents, to locate objects in the dark, and to provide an early warning before being hit in the face with a flying object.

The Respiratory System

Some dogs, like the bloodhound, are bred and used for their keen sense of smell. These animals are instrumental in finding lost people in woods, over mountains, etc., with only the scent of the owner on a piece of clothing to go by.

With 40 times more smell-sensitive receptors than humans have, dogs have an extremely sensitive sense of smell of scents. These receptors are also used by the dog for social interactions.

The nostrils of a dog's nose are used to determine the direction of where the scent is coming from. The dog uses approximately 3-7 sniffs to bring the odor into his nose and the scent molecules accumulate in the nasal chambers. Each additional sniff that the dog makes increases the intensity of the odor, or scent. This is how a dog can identify even the slightest amount of odor (like drugs in a suitcase at the airport).

A dog's nose is slightly wet to the touch. This is because the dog's wet nose, or rhimarium, is used to determine in what direction the air is blowing in the odor. There are cold receptors in the skin that react to the cooling off of the skin through evaporation of air moisture currents.

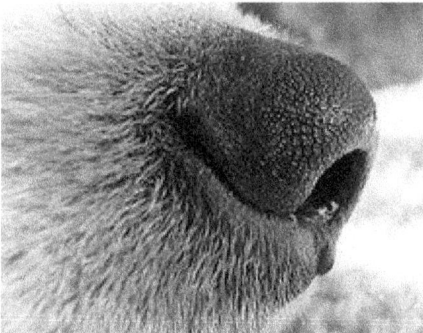

www.Wikipedea.com(2018)

The Dog's Nose

Panting

A dog is able to regulate its body temperature through panting (which is when you see an animal's tongue hanging out of their mouth), and also through the sweating of their paws.

By panting, canines can move cooler air over the moist surfaces of their tongues and lungs and exhale the warmer air from their bodies. A set of nasal turbinates in the nasal cavities allow for heat exchange between small arteries and veins in canines. Cats have nasal turbinates too, but theirs are mostly smaller and less developed than a dog's. This structure also adds the canine in conserving water when in arid conditions which allows the canine to survive in conditions which are very dry and/or very cold such as in the Artic. (Think of the dogs that pull sleds there).

Lungs

In canines, the respiratory system includes a set or organs that are responsible for gas exchange and cellular respiration. The main function of the respiratory system is to first absorb oxygen, and then to eliminate it (carbon dioxide) from the body.

The system also plays an important part in the thermoregulation of the animal because, unlike humans, dogs have only a few sweat glands on their skin. But like humans, they can sweat through their paws (feet and hands for humans).

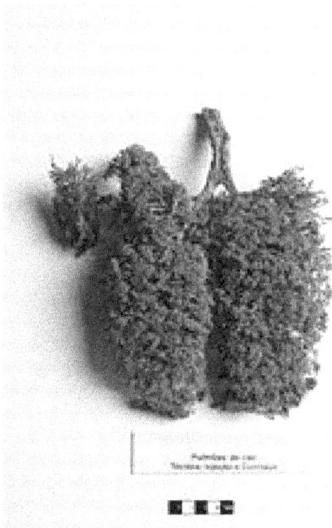

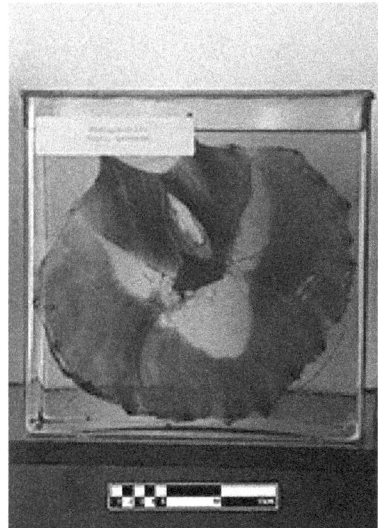

Dog Lungs (left) and Diaphragm (right)
(images taken from www.wikipedea.com 2018)

In the previous picture, you can see what the dog lungs and diaphragm look like. On the left is the picture of the dog's lungs which you can see contains two large lungs and lobes. The lungs have a spongy appearance and what looks like branches, which are actually delicate bronchioles. At the end of each branch is a closed, thin-walled chamber called the alveoli where the gas exchange takes place.

In the previous picture, you can see what the dogs diaphragm looks like (picture on the right). The diaphragm is a muscular structure that divides the peritoneal cavity and the pleural cavity and assists the ribs during the inhalation.

Antibacterial-peppermint, lemongrass, thyme CT thymol
Antiviral-eucalyptus, ginger, Niaouli, ravensara, black pepper
Expectorant-turmeric, eucalyptus, ginger, rosemary
Antispasmodic-clary sage, petitgrain, marjoram, basil, tarragon, frankincense
Decongestant-eucalyptus, rosemary, cardamom, spike lavender

Common Pathogens

Disease/Ailment	Description
Asthma	Chronic inflammatory disease causes swelling in the bronchial tubes or lining of the trachea
Bronchitis	Inflammation of a bronchus
Bronchogenic carcinoma	Malignant tumor originating in the bronchi. Also called Lung Cancer.
Chronic obstructive disease (COPD)	Progressive, chronic groups of pulmonary conditions with obstruction of air through the airways.
Common cold	Viral infection that causes nasal congestion, etc..
Croup	Acute respiratory condition with a barking cough
Deviated septum	Nasal septum strays from the midline of the nasal cavity
Emphysema	Ruptured alveoli in the lungs make breathing difficult
Epistaxis	A nosebleed
IRDS	Disease characterized by lack of surfactant in the alveoli
Laryngitis	Inflammation of the mucous lining of the larynx
Pharyngitis	Inflammation or infection of the pharynx
Pneumonia	Acute inflammation of the lungs
Rhinitis	Inflammation of the nasal mucosa
Tuberculosis	Chronic bacillus infection affecting the lungs

The Integumentary System (skin)

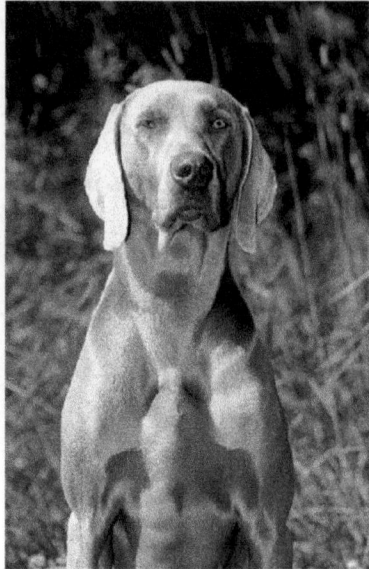

The largest organ of the body, the skin is the body's protection against heat, light, dehydration and pathogens. The skin regulates the heat in the body, secretes perspiration to cool the body and sebum to lubricate the skin, it excretes wastes and absorbs Vitamin D for the body to use.

The skin also has appendages which include the hair, nails and the skin gland. These appendages, along with the skin itself as the principal organ, are all part of the integumentary system. The functions of the integumentary system include:

Protection-The skin forms a barrier to ward against invading and harmful pathogens such as viruses and bacteria. It also protects internal organs from harmful ultraviolet rays.

Regulation-The skin allows us to sweat when we are hot in order to allow evaporation to cool us. Superficial blood vessels constrict to warm us. And a layer of fat (lipids) offers us a layer of insulation.

Sensory reception-The skin has millions of sensory receptors that can detect pain, touch, pressure, temperature, etc. and send these messages to the brain and spinal cord to act on. (Like to remove your hand from a fire).

Wound and Tissue Repair

Skin goes through three separate phases in order to accomplish tissue and wound repair. These phases are: inflammation, regeneration and remodeling.

Coat

In canines, appendages of hair to the skin can be referred to as the dog's coat.

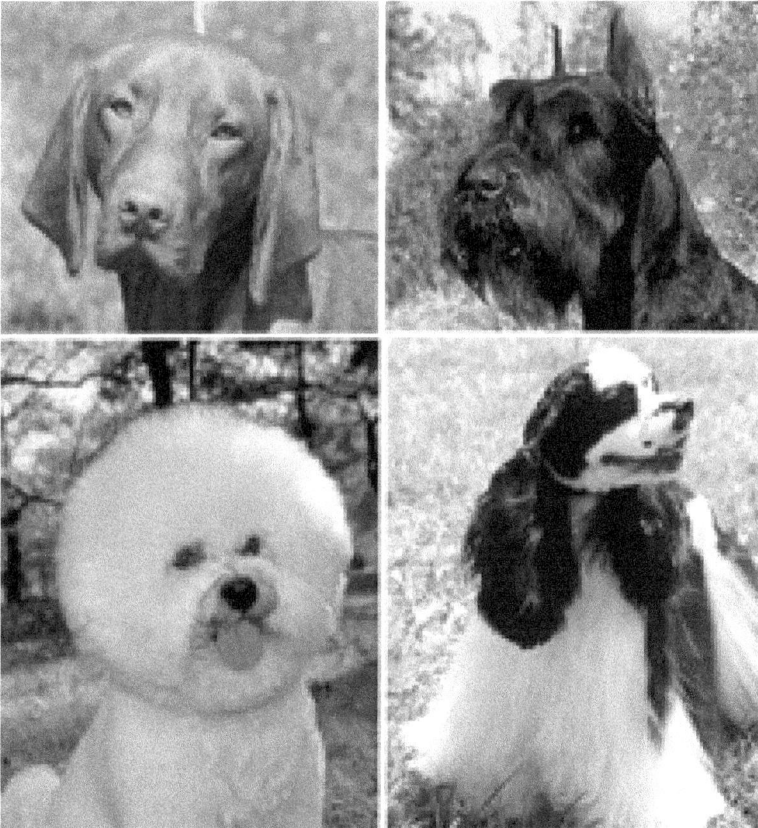

Coat Variations
(images from www.wikipedea.com 2018)

Today's dogs exhibit a varied array of fur coats (or lack thereof). These coats have different color, markings and texture. Just like in people, a therapist can tell the health of a person by looking at the color, texture and markings on the human skin, so too can a vet tell what is going on with an animal by looking at its coat.

Since a dogs coat is make up of mostly protein and amino acids, you can see tell when a dog is lacking good nutrition when they have a dull coat. The fur can also shelter unwanted guests such as fleas, tics and parasites that can lead to infections and discomfort. A cost should have a slight shine in it to show that it is healthy. Good grooming habits and consistent inspection is important to maintaining the health of your pet. Believe it or not, a good hairdresser can also tell the health of her human client through the hair.

If your pet is losing patches of its coat hair, or is bald, it can be a sign of such problems such as tumors, infestation, cancer, and stress.

The 'smell' test

After you have given your dog a bath, look and feel its coat. It should smell fresh and feel clean.

Strong musky, or foul odor-May indicate bacterial infection, fungus, fleas, or dry skin

Chronic foul smelling fur-May indicate a serious condition. Vet visit is suggested.

Tail

There are almost as many different shapes of dog tails as there are breeds. Some dogs have a gland on the dorsal (upper) surface of their tail. This gland is called the violet, or supracaudal gland. This is an important gland for certain mammals such as badgers, wolves, foxes, cats, and dogs as it contains sweat glands and sebaceous glands.

The animals use these glands to signal, or scent mark, their territory. To mark their territory, the animal will secrete a mixture that is a blend of volatile terpenes.

In some dogs, the violet, or supracaudal gland is completely absent, but for those dogs that have one, the gland is located above the 9th caudal vertebra. The violet gland secretes protein and hydrophobic lipids and plays a role in steroid hormone metabolism.

Footpad

The footpad of a dog contains a blood system that is able to recirculate heat in the dog's body. This helps the animal stand on surfaces such as snow or ice for long periods of time. The system is able to bring blood to the footpad and retain it there in the pad surface.

Essential oils can be used for scar and wound healing, burns, dermatitis, eczema, psoriasis, and more through topical uses in massage, baths, and compresses.

Anti-inflammatory-lavender, chamomile, rose, yarrow

Cicatrizants-lavender, rose, frankincense, g. chamomile, myrrh, helichrysum, neroli

Scars-lavandin, lavender, ginger, black pepper, rosemary

Burns-lavender, g. chamomile, peppermint

Dermatitis and Eczema-mandarin, geranium, palmarosa, rose, calendula

Psoriasis-lavender, german chamomile, rose, palmarosa, calendula, mandarin, helichrysum, neroli, blue cypress

Anti-pruritics-lavender, tea tree, peppermint

Moisturizers-german chamomile, mandarin, rose, geranium, palmarosa

Pancreas-g. chamomile, coriander, dill, cinnamon, and cypress

Ovaries-clary sage, helichrysum, frankincense, geranium, cypress, lavender

Testes/Gonads-r. chamomile, lavender, rosemary

Common Pathogens

Disease/Ailment	Description
Acne	Inflammatory condition of the sebaceous glands and hair follicles resulting in pimples, cysts, blackheads, etc.
Basal cell carcinoma	Cancerous tumor of the epidermis from sun exposure
Burns	Injury to skin tissue by heat, fire, chemicals, etc.
Cellulitis	Cute infection and inflammation of the skin
Dermatitis	Inflammation of the skin
Eczema	Inflammation of the epidermis with red, itchy lesions
Folliculitis	Inflammation of the hair follicles with pustules
Furnucle	Bacterial infection of a hair follicle with pain. A boil.
Gangrene	Tissue necrosis usually due to deficient blood supply
Herpes	Small, painful blisters caused by herpes virus
Kaposi's sarcoma	Skin cancer often seen in AIDS
Malignant melanoma	Skin cancer that spreads to the internal organs
Nevus	Pigmented elevated spot on the surface of the skin (mole)
Psoriasis	Chronic inflammatory condition with crusty lesions
Purpura	Hemorrhages in the skin due to fragile blood vessels
Rubella	Contagious viral skin infections with rash and fever
Scabies	Contagious skin disease with itching, blisters and pustules
Shingles	Rash and pain that erupts along nerve paths of the body
Squamous cell carcinoma (SCC)	Epidermal cancer resulting in a crusted nodule that ulcerates and bleeds
Tinea	Fungal skin disease with itchy, scaly lesions and rash

Urticaria	Skin eruption of pale red itchy wheal. (hives)
Vitiligo	Lack of pigment in areas of the skin causing white appearance. Whole body vitiligo is referred to as albino.
Warts	Benign growth with rough surface caused by a virus

The Circulatory (Cardiovascular) System

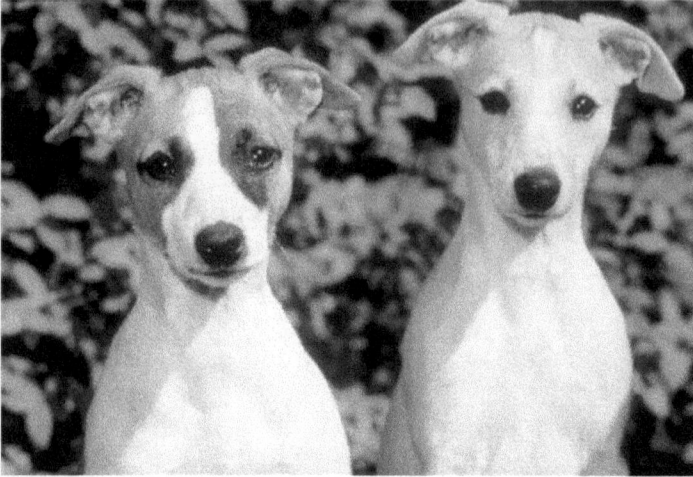

It's the responsibility of the Circulatory (Cardiovascular) System to transport oxygen and nutrients, remove wastes, to regulate the body's temperature, hormone levels and pH of fluids. The heart is the major organ of this system of the body. It contains four chambers, or cavities, that pump and circulate blood through the body and lungs. It weight approximately 9 ounces and is the size of human fist. It is controlled by the autonomic nervous system which means that you don't have to make it pump blood; it does this on its own. It is blood vessels that transports blood away from the heart and back again. There are three major blood vessels: Arteries, veins, and capillaries.

Arteries transport blood away from the heart while veins transport blood back to the heart. The largest artery in the body is called the *aorta*. The walls of the arteries expand during the contraction of the heart and relax between the beats of the heart. When you take a pulse, it reflects the rate of the heart.

Veins have thin walls and transport blood from tissues and the lungs back to the heart again to become filtered. Veins are generally located closer to the surface of the skin are often used to administer intravenous medications (IV) or when you need to have blood drawn.

The *capillaries* are tiny blood vessels with thin walls that serve as exchange vessels. Capillaries send vital oxygen and nutrients to tissues and receive waste products and carbon dioxide in exchange.

Blood is the life line of the body. It is the fluid that transports oxygen from the lungs, nutrients to the cells, hormones from the endocrine system and protects the body from invasion and infection. Blood regulates the pH levels of the body and balances the electrolytes to insure proper cell functioning.

Deoxygenated blood flows from the heart to the lungs where it receives oxygen. From the lungs, oxygenated blood flows back to the heart and out to the body via the aorta.

Blood pressure is the measurement of the force exerted by blood against the walls of the blood vessel. It is measured in two numbers, one placed over the other. The top number is called the systolic pressure (recorded during ventricular contraction) and the bottom number is called the diastolic pressure (recorded during ventricular relaxation. The top number (systolic) should always be higher than the bottom number (diastolic). A normal blood pressure for adults is calculated at 120/80, but a healthy range is anything between 90/60 to 140/90.

Aromatherapy affects the cardiovascular system by increasing local circulation, reducing clotting, reducing high blood pressure through massage, reducing angina and arrhythmia by relaxing and balancing the cardiovascular system. Varicose veins may be helped with essential oils as will bruising and inflammation.

Essential Oils for this system:

Hypotensive-help to lower blood pressure by dilating blood vessels (vasodilation), relaxing the smooth muscle of the vein's walls (vasorelaxation), or increasing parasympathetic nerve activity/decreasing nerve activity. Lavender, celery seed, basil, cedarwood, neroli, spikenard, geranium

Hypertensive-raises blood pressure. Cyprus, lemon, juniper

Rubefacient-Increases local peripheral circulation. Cinnamon, eucalyptus

Anticoagulant-for people who have risks for blood clots. Basil, helichrysum

Varicose veins-cypress, lemon, geranium, peppermint,
palmarosa, helichrysum

Common Pathogens

Disease/Ailment	Description
Anemia	Deficiency of red blood cells in the blood
Aneurysm	Weakness in artery wall causing a sac to form
Angina pectoris	Severe chest pain with constriction around the heart
Angioma	Tumor consisting of blood vessels; usually benign
Arrhythmia	Irregular heartbeat
Arteriosclerosis	Hardening or thickening of the walls of the arteries
Arteritis	Inflammation of an artery
Atherosclerosis	Buildup of fatty substances on the inner walls of the arteries
Cardiomyopathy	Disease that deteriorates the heart muscle
Embolism	Obstruction of a blood vessel by a blood clot or object
Hypertension	High blood pressure
Hypotension	Low blood pressure
Ischemia	Lack of blood supply due to an obstruction
Leukemia	Cancer of the white blood cells
Phlebitis	Inflammation of a vein
Spider veins	Superficial network of veins
Thrombus	Blood clot within a blood vessel
Varicose Veins	Swelling of veins in legs

The Digestive System

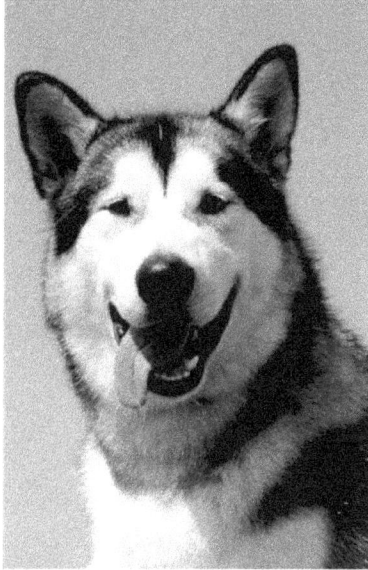

Digestive system

The organs that make up the canine digestive system are:

- Mouth
- Tongue
- Esophagus
- Stomach
- Liver
- Pancreas
- Large intestine
- Small intestine
- Rectum
- Anus
- Dog cecum
- Dog digestive tract
- Dog ileum

A dog eats and processes food differently than a human's body which is the reason that we must be so careful when using essential oils on our pets.

The Mouth

A dog's mouth is used for biting and chewing large pieces of food. The jaws and teeth ingest meat, bones and fat products.

Esophagus to Stomach

Food passes from the dog's mouth through the esophagus to the stomach. Once there, the food is processed with hydrochloric acid to break down of the large pieces of food. If the food that is ingested is not processed correctly, the dog will naturally regurgitate it, and then swallow it.

Stomach to Small Intestine

From the stomach, processed food (now a liquid) will pass through to the small intestine where the nutrients from the food will be assimilated into the dog's body.

Small Intestine to Large Intestine

Whatever is not assimilated in the small intestine goes on to the large intestine where it will eventually end up as waste and get passed out through the dog's rectum in the form of feces.

Other Considerations

It takes approximately 8-9 hours for food to go through the entire digestive process in an <u>adult</u> dog. This is important to know, as an Aromatherapist, since it will take that long for oils to get processed through the digestive system.

The digestive system of canines can be a good indicator when illness is present. Be familiar with your dog's eating habits and pooping habits. If your dog is bloat or gas, this could indicate a poor diet or something much more serious.

Essential oils that most influence this body system includes: calming, antispasmodic, digestive stimulants, appetite stimulants or suppressers, and hepatics. These oils can be used in enemas, baths, compresses, rubs, heat applications, and massages.

Antispasmodic-peppermint, tarragon, Melissa, cardamom, basil, , rose, roman chamomile
Digestive stimulant-sage, rosemary, fennel
Appetite stimulant-cardamon, lemon, peppermint, bergamot, fennel, tarragon
Constipation-fennel, black pepper, marjoram, ginger
IBS-german chamomile, yarrow, lavender, turmeric, helichrysum, peppermint, rosemary, cardamom, tarragon,

Common Pathogens

Disease/Ailment	Description
Anorexia	Loss of appetite
Anorexia nervosa	Eating disorder involving refusal to eat
Appendicitis	Inflammation of the appendix
Bulimia	Eating disorder characterized by binging then purging
Cholecystitis	Inflammation of the gallbladder caused by gallstones
Cirrhosis	Chronic disease of the liver causing liver dysfunction
Colorectal cancer	Cancers of the colon
Constipation	Difficult or infrequent defecation
Crohn's disease	Chronic inflammatory bowel disease affecting the colon

Diarrhea	Passing of frequent watery bowel movements
Diverticulitis	Inflammation of a diverticulum
Diverticulosis	Condition of having diverticula in the intestinal tract
Dyspepsia	Indigestion
Enteritis	Inflammation of the small intestine
Gastritis	Inflammation of the stomach
Gastroenteritis	Inflammation of the stomach and small intestine
Hemorrhoids	Varicose veins in the rectum
Hepatitis	Inflammation of the liver generally due to viral infection
Hiatal hernia	Abnormal protrusion in the upper portion of the stomach
(IBS) Inflammatory bowel disease	Chronic inflammatory condition with multiple ulcers forming on the mucous membrane of the color.
Inguinal hernia	Abnormal protrusion of a portion of the small intestine
(IBS) Irritable bowel syndrome	Disturbances in intestinal function from unknown causes. Also called spastic colon.
Pancreatic cancer	Cancer of the pancreas
Peptic ulcer disease	Ulcer occurring in the lining of the lower esophagus, stomach or duodenum.
Polyps	Small tumors attached to the mucous membrane of the colon and/or large intestine.
Pyrosis	Painful burning sensation cause by stomach acid. Heartburn.
Volvulus	Painful condition where the bowel twists up on itself.

Musculoskeletal System

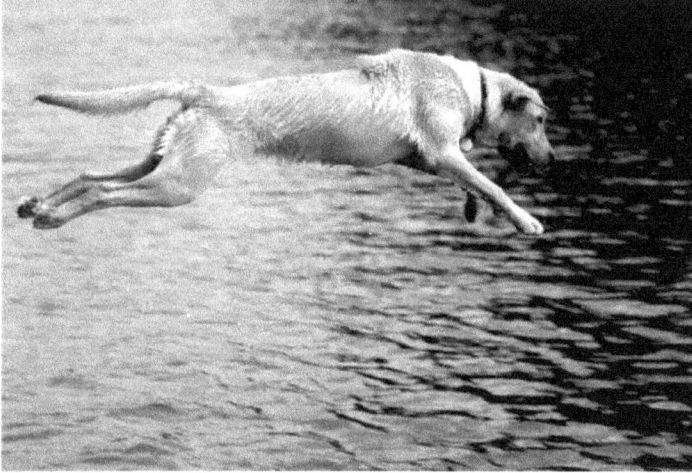

The Musculoskeletal System deals with movement of the body, posture, stability, and holding the bones and joints stable. This system contains the muscles, connective tissues, bones, ligaments, tendons and fascia. There are three major types of muscles: skeletal, smooth and cardiac.

There are hundreds of skeletal muscles in the human body. These muscles are composed of a group of fibers and are held together by connective tissue called *fascia.* Skeletal muscles attach directly or indirectly to bones and overlap joints. These muscles provide for a variety of voluntary body movement by contraction, extension and elasticity.

Smooth muscles are responsible for the involuntary actions of the muscle such as pushing food through the digestive system, uterine contractions, constricting or dilating a blood vessel, etc. They are generally found in the digestive organs, respiratory organs, vascular organs, etc.

Cardiac muscles comprise the wall of the heart and are called *myocardium.* These muscles produce the involuntary actions that cause the heart to pump blood through the chambers and blood vessels. This happens without us thinking about it.

In dogs, the muscles work the same way as they do in humans. Dog muscles are connected to the skeletal system, skin, and other muscles to provide movement and stability. There are voluntary (controlled by conscious thought) and involuntary muscles (controlled by the brain through the autonomic nervous system). Involuntary muscles make the heart pump blood, the lungs breathe air, and takes food through the digestive processes, all without the dog having to think about it.

However, in dogs, the muscles are broken down into two distinct regions: The Thoracic Limb and the Pelvic Limb. The Thoracic Limb consists of all muscles located in the upper trunk of the dog's body and the Pelvic Limb consists of all the muscles located in the lower region.

The Thoracic Limb contains seven major muscles: the supraspinatus, infraspinatus, pectoral, trapezius, biceps brachii, brachialis, and triceps brachii muscles. The Pelvic Limb contains seven muscles, or muscle groups: the gluteal muscle, biceps femoris, semitendinosus, semimembranosus, quadriceps femoris, cranial tibial muscles, and Achilles tendon. The Pelvic Limb is responsible for the support and movement of the hip muscles and joints.

There are many diseases, ailments and disorders that are specifically associated with the muscular system. On the following page is a small list of some of those pathogens.

Methods of Application

Essential oils can affect the muscles of the body by absorption through the skin, compresses, internally and topically. You can apply (massage or by compresses) essential oils to affected areas of the body to increase circulation, to cool, as an anti-inflammatory, analgesic for pain relief, antispasmodic (for stomach cramping, etc.)

Methods of application for this system include cold and hot compresses for sprains and strains, arthritis joints, aching muscles, cramps and spasms. Baths using essential oils and massaging with essential oils can help with muscles strains and sprains, knotted muscles, Fibromyalgia and for overuse injuries. This includes stress, TMJ, and tension headaches.

Analgesic-bay laurel, black pepper, chamomile,
    lavender, lavandin, peppermint,
Anti-inflammatory (*cooling*)-blue cypress, chamomile,
    helichrysum, lavender, palmarosa, turmeric, yarrow
Anti-inflammatory (*warming*)-black pepper, clover, cardamom,
    cumin, ginger, nutmeg
Antispasmodic-basil, black pepper, cardamom, clary sage,
    lavender, marjoram, petitgrain, r. chamomile
Arthritis-spike lavender, bay laurel, ginger, cardamom
Gout-lavender, peppermint, g. chamomile, helichrysum, yarrow,
    carrot, juniper
Scleroderma-calendula rose hip, sandalwood, rose, palmarosa,
    rock rose, geranium
Fibromyalgia-bay laurel, black pepper, ginger
Cramps and Spasms-marjoram, basil, cardamom, sage, r.
    chamomile, tarragon
TMJ-wintergreen, marjoram, black pepper, basil, g. chamomile.
Tension Headaches-lavender, basil, rosemary, r. chamomile,
    peppermint

Common Pathogens

Disease/Ailment	Description
Adhesion	Built up of layers of fascial tissue
Atrophy	Loss of muscle mass/strength due to immobility
Bursitis	Inflammation of a bursa
Contracture	Shortening of muscle fibers, tendons or fascia
Cramps	Involuntary and painful muscle twitch (spasm)
Fibromyalgia	Chronic condition of pain and aching muscles- 18 points
Hernia	Tear in muscle wall that allows an organ to protrude
Muscular Dystrophy (MS)	Chronic, genetic diseases causing muscles to degenerate and weaken ending in atrophy
Myasthenia gravis	Autoimmune muscle disease causing weakness/fatigue
Repetitive Motion Disorder	Damage to joints, muscles, etc. due to repetitive motions.
Scar Tissue	Collagen fibers laid down over areas of injury in muscle
Spasms	Sudden and violent muscle contraction. A cramp.
Sprain	Acute injury to ligaments around joints (whiplash)
Strains	Injury or tear in muscle, tendon and attachments to bone
Tendinitis	Inflammation of a tendon after repetitive movements
Tetanus	Bacterial disease causing locking of the jaw
TMJ	Muscle contraction of the jaw

The Skeletal System

The skeleton provides the dog the ability to run, jump and leap.

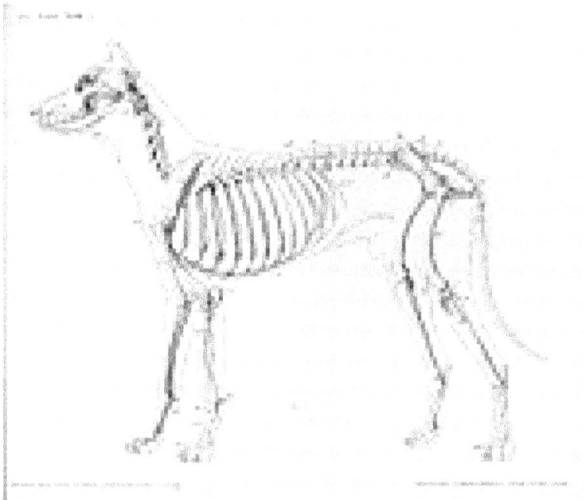

Transferred from de.wikipedia to Commons File:Dog anatomy lateral skeleton view.jpg

The skeleton system contains the following number of bones, or vertebraes:

A – Cervical or Neck Bones (7 in number). (Humans have 7 also)

B – Dorsal or Thoracic Bones (13 in number, each bearing a rib). (Humans have 12)

C – Lumbar Bones (7 in number). (Humans have 7)

D – Sacral Bones (3 in number). (Humans have 5 that fuse into 1)

E – Caudal or Tail Bones (20 to 23 in number). (Humans have 1 that is called the Cocyx, or tailbone).

In the preceding image of the skeleton of a dog, the following are the word labels that go with the image.

1 – Cranium, or Skull.
2 – Maxilla.
3 – Mandible, or Lower jaw .
4 – Atlas.
5 – Axis.
6 – Scapula, or Shoulder-blade.
7 – Spine of scapula.
8 – Humerus.
9 – Radius.
10 – Ulna.
11 – Phalanges.
12 – Metacarpal Bones.
13 – Carpal Bones or Wrist-bones.
14 – Sternum, or Breast-bone.
15 – Cartilaginous part of rib.
16 – Ribs (13 in number).
17 – Phalanges.
18 – Metatarsal Bones.
19 – Tarsal Bones.
20 – Calcaneus (os calcu).
21 – Fibula.
22 – Tibia.
23 – Patella, or Knee-cap.
24 – Femur.
25 – Ischium.
26 – Pelvis, or Hip-bone.

In humans, the skeletal system is the support of the human body. Through this system, hair, skin and nails are all affected. There are 206 bones in the adult human body that store minerals, protect vital organs, and allow movement of the body to occur. Additional parts of the skeleton include cartilage, tendons, ligaments and joints. A dog's body, in comparison has 319-321 bones (115 more than humans).

Common Pathogens

Disease/Ailment	Description
Arthritis	Inflammation of a joint
Bunion	Inflammation of the bursa of the big toe
Carpal Tunnel	Compression of the nerve and ligaments of the wrist
Fracture	Broken bone
Ganglion cyst	Fluid-filled synovial sacks found on joint capsules and tendons
Gout	Inflammation of the joints caused by excessive uric acid in the body
Myeloma	Malignant tumor of the bone marrow
Osteoarthritis	Degeneration of bones and joint due to arthritis
Osteporosis	Loss of bone density and thinning of bone tissue
Rheumatoid arthritis	Autoimmune disorder with inflammation of joints
Spondylosis	Degenerative condition of the vertebrae column
Sprain	Damage to the ligaments surrounding a joint due to overstretching
Whiplash	Injury to the cervical spine due to violent movement

Essential oils can help bones that are inflamed or in pain. Essential oils for this system include lavender, chamomile, helichrysum, cypress, juniper and grapefruit

Essential Oils for Arthritis and Arthritic Pain

Essential Oil	Function
Basil	Good for arthritis and rheumatism, muscle spasm and gout.
Cedarwood	Decongests the lymph system, unblocks arteries, breaks down fat deposits, and improves poor circulation. Reduces fluid retention.
Clove Bud	Analgesic (pain relief). Arthritis and muscle cramps.
Eucalyptus	Reduces fluid retention. Eases muscle aches and rheumatism
Fennel	Good for lymph and fluid retention. Improves circulation.
Frankincense	Relieves muscle aches and pain caused by rheumatism. Helps anxiety, asthma, bronchitis, stress, scars and stretch marks.
Geranium	Reduces fluid retention, balances hormones, and eases anxiety, depression and nervous tension. Stimulates circulation.
Lavender	Good for headaches, insomnia and inflammation.
Lemon	Cleanse and detoxify. Makes the body more alkaline helping arthritis, gout, rheumatism, pain and inflammation of the joints.
Lemongrass	Boosts the immune system, tones muscles, relieves tired aching legs and eliminates lactic acid build-up. Tendons, ligaments
Palmarosa	Anti-viral and Anti-fungal. Cellular stimulant, relieves stiff and sore muscles, uplifting and stress reducing.
Peppermint	Cooling and Pain relieving. Good for headaches and pain in general. Great for muscular aches and pains. Inflammation

Rosemary	Warming oil aids in stimulating the circulatory system and tones muscles. Rub into joints to ease pain. Reduces cellulite, gout pain, fatigue, and fluid retention.
Helichrysum	Inflammation, muscle cramps, arthritis
Pepper	Inflammation
Hyssop	Inflammation

The Immune System
The main responsibility of the Immune System is to identify foreign invaders and neutralize them. The immune system includes the digestive system, integumentary system, cardiovascular system, endocrine system and the lymphatic system. The cells of the immune system are called *lymphocytes*. Lymphocytes are broken down into two major cells-the B cells and T-cells and are manufactured in the bone marrow. The T-cells, and a subgroup called *killer cells*, are created to fight invading pathogens. Pathogens include everything from viruses and bacteria to parasitic worms and cancer.

Disorders of the immune system include autoimmune diseases (Hashimoto's thyroiditis), inflammatory diseases (rheumatoid arthritis), and immunodeficiency (HIV/AIDS). Addition ailments include diabetes, and lupus.

Essential oils can help boost the immunity system by reducing stress levels and calming the nervous system. Oils can also help with autoimmune disease, allergies, hives, rashes, chronic fatigue and viral illnesses. Essential oils can help boost the immunity system by reducing stress levels and calming the nervous system. Oils can also help with autoimmune disease, allergies, hives, rashes, chronic fatigue and viral illnesses.

There are two functional divisions of the immune system (innate and adaptive). The innate immune system is the dog's first line of defense and comes in the form of the skin, stomach acid, saliva and respiratory system. The adaptive immune system kicks in to action once foreign invaders have entered the body. This occurs through the monocytes and macrophages, etc. And this system will remember the invaders in case it ever returns again in the future. Dogs can also suffer from an autoimmune disease such as:

Juvenile diabetes (Organ Specific)
Pemphigus vulgaris (a skin condition)
Myasthenia gravis (a nerve condition)
Autoimmune hemolytic anemia
Rheumatoid arthritis
Polymyositis (a muscle condition)
Systemic lupus erythematosis (SLE)

In the immune system, aromatherapy can be used in two ways. One way is to oppose the threatening pathogens by using essential oils that are antiviral or antibacterial. Another way to use essential oils is to increase the activity and strengthen the organ and cells that are under attack.

Antibacterial- clove, basil, oregano, thyme
Antiviral- marjoram, lavender, peppermint, eucalyptus,
        sandalwood, lemongrass
Antifungal-lemongrass, Melissa, eucalyptus, geranium, clove,
        patchouli, petitgrain, spearmint
Depressed Immunity-bay laurel, frankincense, marjoram,
        palmarosa, lemongrass, geranium, patchouli
Chronic Fatigue-Black spruce, pine, ginger, rosemary,
        cardamom, frankincense
Allergies-chamomile, cedar, turmeric, lavender
Candidiasis-geranium, patchouli, palmarosa
Viral Infections-eucalyptus, marjoram, ravensara, ginger,
        cardamon

Use the following essential oils to build up the strength of the following organs:

Spleen-black pepper, lavender
Adrenal Gland-rosemary, geranium

NOTE: If you have depleted your immune system it may take you at least one month of use before you start to feel better. It does take time to strengthen a weakened immune system because there are so many systems involved in the process and you must consider these other systems when deciding on what oils to use and how to use them.

Common Pathogens

Disease/Ailment	Description
Adhesion	Built up of layers of fascial tissue
Atrophy	Loss of muscle mass/strength due to immobility
Bursitis	Inflammation of a bursa
Contracture	Shortening of muscle fibers, tendons or fascia
Cramps	Involuntary and painful muscle twitch (spasm)
Fibromyalgia	Chronic condition of pain and aching muscles-18 points
Hernia	Tear in muscle wall that allows an organ to protrude
Muscular Dystrophy (MS)	Chronic, genetic diseases causing muscles to degenerate and weaken ending in atrophy
Myasthenia gravis	Autoimmune muscle disease causing weakness/fatigue
Repetitive Motion Disorder	Damage to joints, muscles, etc. due to repetitive motions.
Scar Tissue	Collagen fibers laid down over areas of injury in muscle
Spasms	Sudden and violent muscle contraction. A cramp.
Sprain	Acute injury to ligaments around joints (whiplash)
Strains	Injury or tear in muscle, tendon and attachments to bone
Tendinitis	Inflammation of a tendon after repetitive movements
Tetanus	Bacterial disease causing locking of the jaw
TMJ	Muscle contraction of the jaw

The Urinary System

The Urinary System is responsible for making urine, filtering and removing waste products, adjusting water and electrolytes levels and maintaining the correct pH levels in the body. Not only is this system responsible for processing Vitamin D, it is also responsible for the production of hormones called erythropoietin and renin which help to maintain blood pressure, and produce blood cells.

In dogs, the urinary system, or urinary tract, includes the kidneys, the ureters, the bladder, and the urethra.

Problems that can affect a dog's lower urinary System.

- Bladder inflammation or infection
- Incontinence from excessive water drinking or weak bladder/hormonal issue
- Trauma
- Cancer
- Stress
- Spinal cord abnormalities
- Congenital abnormality
- Prostate disease
- Stones, crystals or debris

The most common problems are often seen in dogs that are over the age of seven. These problems usually include incontinence (due to weak urinary sphincter muscle), bacterial infections, endocrine diseases, and diabetes mellitus. Below are listed some signs to look for to see if your pet may have problems:

- Fever
- Bloody or cloudy urine
- Inability to urinate
- Lethargy
- Vomiting

- Frequent urination
- Straining to urinate
- Painful urination
- Frequent licking
- Soiling
- Strong urine odor
- Weight loss
- Increased water consumption
- Pain, irritability

Terms of the Urinary System:

Urination or Voiding-passage of urine from the body or the emptying of the bladder.

Enuresis-involuntary urination (bed wetting)

Anuria-absence of urine

Oliguria-scanty amounts of urine

Polyuria-large amount of urine

Renal failure- Kidneys cannot clear blood of urea or waste products. Toxic condition occurs.

Urinary incontinence- Leakage of urine caused by age and weakened sphincter muscles.

Uremia-Terminal stage of renal failure

Essential oils to use for the urinary tract infection include those to help in the elimination of excess fluid in the body, those that stimulate the circulatory and lymphatic systems of the body and those that help with inflammation, irritation and pain. Methods of application include Sitz baths, baths, compresses, and massage oils.

Analgesic-R. chamomile, peppermint, lavender, marjoram
Antimicrobial-Frankincense, bergamot, lemon, thyme linalol
Antibacterial-peppermint, lemongrass, thyme CT thymol
Anti-inflammatory-R. chamomile, lavender sandalwood.

Antiviral-eucalyptus, ginger, Niaouli, ravensara, black pepper
Antispasmodic-clary sage, petitgrain, marjoram, basil, tarragon,
    frankincense

Urinary Tract Infection: lavender, geranium, myrrh, and sandalwood
    can be used in an abdominal and low-back massage or used in
    baths.

Common Pathogens

Disease/Ailment	Description
Cystitis	Inflammation of the bladder due to bacteria
Glomerulonephritis	Inflammation of the kidneys
Kidney stones	Deposits of calculi (mineral salts) in the kidneys
Polycystic kidney	Formation of noncancerous cysts in the kidneys
Pyelonephritis	Infection of the kidney and renal pelvis
Urinary tract infection (UTI)	Infection of any organ of the urinary system.

The Reproductive System

In male dogs, the Reproductive System includes the penis, bulbus glandis, prepuce,

In female doges, the Reproductive System includes vagina, ovaries, eggs, mammary glands, vulva, fallopian tubes,

In both male and female dogs, puberty occurs between the ages of 6 to 12 months, later in some breeds. The Female dog cycle includes the Proestrus (where eggs in the ovaries mature), the Estrus (where mature eggs are released from ovaries and copulation will result in pregnancy), pregnancy can occur as soon as the first estrus cycle occurs. This time is called "in heat" and can last 5 to 9 days.

It takes an average of 2-4 weeks for the reproduction cycle of the female dog. If mating was successful, then a pregnant female will move to the Diestrus Stage which lasts just under 2 months where progesterone levels are high, mammary glands produce milk. In non-pregnant females, this stage will last 2 to over 3 months.

The last stage of the reproduction cycle is called the Anestrus and this is where the female has no attraction to the male which can last anywhere from four to five months.

The process begins with the male dog sniffing the female dog's vulva for receptivity. If the female is not receptive, she may snap or otherwise move away from the male dog. If the female is receptive, then she will hold her tail to the side in what is called "flagging" so that she allows the male dog to use his penis to penetrate her. The male penis goes in soft and swells while inside. Once locked inside the female, copulation commences which may take anywhere from seconds to 20 minutes, or even longer in some cases.

Gestation takes approximately 2 months from day of ovulation. It is said that if count the teats on the female dog, she will produce half the many offspring. While this may be true for wild animals, it is not so true for domesticated animals due to breeders who expect larger litters for a larger return on their money.

Since the average female dog has 10 teats, the average size of a litter would be five to six puppies. Of course this will depends upon the size, breed, age, and health of the dog. Small dogs tend to have three to four puppies and large breeds may have seven to fifteen puppies. The very young and the very old animals tend to have smaller litter sizes.

Essential oils for this body system:

Essential oils often used to help this body system include antispasmodics for cramping and distressing oils for stress and tensions

Calming-rose, lavender, linden blossom, sandalwood, neroli,r. chamomile, patchouli, bitter orange

Estrogenic-aniseed, geranium, fennel, sage, lemongrass, Melissa

Anti-spasmodic-basil, cardamom, ginger, black pepper, clove, marjoram, rosemary, clary sage, fennel

Emmonagogues-basil, rosemary, juniper, fennel, peppermint, sage, thyme

Dysmenorrhea-r. chamomile, ginger, black pepper, peppermint

PMS-aniseed, geranium, frankincense, fennel, sage, melissa, sandalwood

Urinary Tract Infection-lavender, geranium, sandalwood

Edema-geranium, cypress

Stretch Marks-lavender, mandarin, helichrysum, neroli

Postnatal Depression-rose, marjoram

Leg Cramps-petitgrain, marjoram, black pepper, clary sage, lavender

Morning Sickness-ginger, peppermint

Constipation-ginger, black pepper, rosemary, fennel

Varicose Veins-cypress, geranium

Common Pathogens

Disease/Ailment	Description
Breast cancer	Malignant tumor of the breast
Cervical cancer	Malignant growth in the cervix caused by the human pupilloma virus (HPV). Sexually transmitted virus.
Cryptorchidism	Undescended testes
Dysmenorrhea	Painful cramping with menses
Erectile dysfunction	Failure to achieve erection of the penis
Endometrial cancer	Cancer of the endometrial lining of the uterus
Fibrocystic breast disease	Benign cysts form in the breasts
Fibroid Tumor	Benign fibrous growth occurring in the uterus
Hydrocele	Accumulation of watery fluid in the socrum
Hypospadias	Urethra opens on underside of glans or shaft
Inguinal hernia	Protrusion of abdominopelvic organs
Mastitis	Inflammation of the breasts
Memorrhagia	Excessive bleeding during menses
Ogligospermia	Low sperm production
Ovarian cancer	Cancer of the ovary
Ovarian cyst	Cyst developing in the ovary
Paraphimosis	Foreskin cannot be replaced to usual position after it has been retracted behing the glans
Pelvic inflammatory disease (PID)	Inflammation of the female reproductive organs
Phimosis	Tight foreskin cannot be retracted over glans
Preeclampsia	Toxemia of pregnancy resulting in hypertension, headaches and edema.
Premenstrual syndrome (PMS)	Problems that occur 1-2 weeks before menses that include bloating, headaches, edema, depression, etc.
Prolapsed uterus	Fallen uterus that may cause the cervix to protrude through the vaginal opening
Prostate cancer	Malignancy of the prostate tissue
Testicular cancer	Cancer of the testes

Chapter Seven
Therapeutics

Pharmacologic Properties

Essential oils contain certain properties that make them medicinal in nature. Recent studies have shown great success in using essential oils to prevent the transmission of some staphylococcus, streptococcus and candida.

Some of the medicinal ingredients in plants include menthol, capsaicin, anise and camphor. Essential oils containing these ingredients work on the upper respiratory system of the body and act as mild expectorants, decongestants and antitussives (Capable of relieving or suppressing coughing). Some oils have a diuretic effect (juniper), eugenol effect (clove oil to numb tooth aches), or antiseptic effects (thymol).

Materia Medica

Materia medica is a Latin term that means a collection of knowledge about the therapeutic properties of substances used for healing. Homeopathy has its own material medica. The term was believed to have been first used in the 1st century AD by the Greek physician Pedanius Dioscorides in his writings, *De material medica* (on medical materials). Today, the words '*material medica*' have been replaced by the word, pharmacology. Pharmacology is the science of drugs (their composition, uses, and effects) as it is concerned with medicine and healing. It is also the study of the preparation, properties, uses and actions of drugs, as well as, their interactions with living organisms.

Actions

On the next page is information that I retrieved from www.wikipedia.com on the antimicrobial properties of 21 essential oils and two plant essences. The chart below shows how these oils and plant essences stood up against five food-borne pathogens.

Pharmacology: major drug groups	
Gastrointestinal tract/ metabolism (A)	stomach acid , Antacids H_2 antagonists Proton pump inhibitors Antiemetics, Laxatives Antidiarrhoeals/Antipropulsives Anti-obesity drugs Anti-diabetics Vitamins and Dietary minerals
Blood and blood forming organs (B)	Antithrombotics Antiplatelets Anticoagulants Thrombolytics/fibrinolytics Antihemorrhagics Platelets Coagulants Antifibrinolytics
Cardiovascular system (C)	*cardiac therapy/antianginals* Cardiac glycosides Antiarrhythmics Cardiac stimulants Antihypertensives Diuretics Vasodilators Beta blockers Calcium channel blockers *renin-angiotensin system* ACE inhibitors Angiotensin II receptor antagonists Renin inhibitors Antihyperlipidemics Statins Fibrates Bile acid sequestrants
Skin (D)	Emollients Cicatrizants

	Antipruritics Antipsoriatics Medicated dressings
Genitourinary system (G)	Hormonal contraception Fertility agents SERMs Sex hormones
Endocrine system (H)	Hypothalamic-pituitary hormones Corticosteroids Glucocorticoids Mineralocorticoids Sex hormones Thyroid hormones/Antithyroid agents
Infections and infestations (J, P, QI)	Antimicrobials: Antibacterials (Antimycobacterials) Antifungals, Antivirals Antiparasitics Antiprotozoals Anthelmintics Ectoparasiticides IVIG, Vaccines
Malignant disease (L01-L02)	Anticancer agents Antimetabolites Alkylating Spindle poisons Antineoplastic Topoisomerase inhibitors
Immune disease (L03-L04)	Immunomodulators Immunostimulants Immunosuppressants
Muscles, bones, and joints (M)	Anabolic steroids Anti-inflammatories , NSAIDs Antirheumatics Corticosteroids Muscle relaxants Bisphosphonates
Brain and	Analgesics

nervous system (N)	Anesthetics, General, Local Anorectics Anti-ADHD Agents Antiaddictives Anticonvulsants Antidementia Agents Antidepressants Antimigraine Agents Antiparkinson's Agents Antipsychotics Anxiolytics Depressants Entactogens, Entheogens Euphoriants Hallucinogens, Psychedelics Dissociatives Deliriants Hypnotics/Sedatives Mood Stabilizers Neuroprotectives Nootropics Neurotoxins Orexigenics Serenics Stimulants Wakefulness-Promoting Agents
Respiratory system (R)	Decongestants Bronchodilators Cough medicines H_1 antagonists
Sensory organs (S)	Ophthalmologicals Otologicals
Other ATC (V)	Antidotes Contrast media Radiopharmaceuticals Dressings

Chapter Eight
Safety

Because essential oils have pharmacological benefits to them, they should be used and handled with care. Some essential oils are applied directly to the skin, some are inhaled and others are used on pets, or for cooking. Some oils can cause allergic reactions when applied to skin of both humans and animals, so these should be used with care. Oils that can cause allergic reaction over time are called photosensitive, photosensitizers, or skin sensitive. Oils that may prove harmful over long usage, and in fact, may result in a toxic build-up in the liver, is called hepatoxic.

Essential oils (outside of Lavender and Tea Tree) should ever be applied directly from the bottle to the skin. This is called Neat. Before applying essential oils to the skin, they should be mixed with carrier oils such as olive oil, sweet almond oil, etc. We will cover some basic dilution ratios in the chapters to come.

Great care should be taken when giving essential oils to women who are pregnant or nursing, children, pets, people with high or low blood pressure and those who are epileptic or suffer from seizures. Please refer to the list of contraindication before giving certain essentials to your family or clients.

Handling

Since essential oils can be hazardous to specific groups of people, I am sure to wear gloves when I work with them. Since essential oils can be absorbed by the skin, I am sure to be cautious about what essentials, and how much of it, that I allow to be absorbed into my skin. This is especially important to massage therapists who use essential oils in their lotions and creams and massage several clients in one day, day after day. Therapists are absorbing these substances into their body on a daily basis. Wouldn't it be advantageous for them to know what risks they are also taking on?

It is also important to use glass containers and syringes when working with essential oils. Avoid rubbers and plastics as some oils can degrade those materials. The best equipment to use is a chemistry syringe that has a seal and piston that wipes off the essential oil from the wall of the pipette. These syringes are more accurate in measuring the amount of oils that you are actually using and because of that, facilitate better quality control.

Skin Testing-The Patch Test

You should never use essential oils directly on your skin, they should be diluted first. One way to test your blend on yourself, or the person who you are making a blend for, is called a **Patch Test**. To perform the Patch Test, you will apply a drop of the oil (mixed with a carrier oil that you created), on the inside of the forearm.

Cover the drop with a simple bandage and wait 24 hours. After the 24 hour waiting period, remove the bandage and see if there was any reaction on the skin. If there was no reaction, this means that you (or your client) is most likely not sensitive to the oil, or blend that you have created.

Note:

Some of the best places to use the Patch Test are on the most sensitive areas of your body which include the inside of the elbow, back of the wrist, or under the arm. If you do suffer from a reaction, wash with the area with soap and water.

Standard Precautions
- General Do's and Don'ts
- Do not take essential oils internally
- Keep essential oils out of the reach of children and pets
- Keep essential oils out of your eyes and mucous membranes
- Always dilute essential oils in a carrier oil (never apply oils directly to your skin)
- Be sure to use 100% pure essential oils.
- People with Epilepsy should avoid such essential oils as rosemary, and sage.
- If you are taking Staten medications-avoid hepatoxic oils such as grapefruit.
- Remember that citrus oils are photosensitive. Stay out of sunlight for 4-5 hours after applying essential oils. Also, avoid tanning beds when using citrus oils.
- People with estrogenic cancers should avoid such essential oils as rose, clary sage and geranium.
- People with high blood pressure, or those who are taking blood thinner, should avoid the oils of cinnamon, sage and hyssop.
- Asthma sufferers should avoid steam inhalation as this may irritate and aggravate the mucus membranes. Avoid essential oil of thyme.
- Avoid prolonged use of essential oils. Have 5-6 days on and take 1-2 days off.
- Avoid the essential oil of pine if you have prostate concerns.
- Store essential oils in colored glass containers out of direct sunlight.
- Be sure to use proper dosages for children and pets-do not use adult dosages.
- Be sure to have proper ventilation when using essential oils over a long period of time.
- Be sure to perform a Patch Test on yourself before applying essential oils to your entire body, especially if you have sensitive skin.

- Always check with your client about their past reactions to using essential oils.
- Refrigerate carrier oils to prevent them from becoming rancid.
- Old oils are more prone to cause skin reactions. Throw these oils out. Some oils like patchouli and sandalwood get better with age-most do not.
- If you keep a bird in your home, stay away from using essential oils in a diffuser.
- Use caution during pregnancy and while nursing. Safe essential oils include lavender, mandarin and Roman Chamomile.

Emergency Issues

What to do for reactions:

If you accidentally ingest an essential oil, call your local Poison Control Center. Do NOT induce vomiting or give liquids to drink.

If a skin reaction or irritation appears, stop using essential oils. Some essential oils like cinnamon, oregano, fennel, clove and verbena can cause skin irritation. The best relief from skin irritations due to essential oils is to apply a fatty oil, such as coconut, which will dilute the essential oil.

If you accidentally get an essential oil in your eye-don't rub it! Instead, soak a cotton ball into milk or vegetable oil and place it in the affected area. You can also try to use coconut oil, olive oil, cooking oil or milk. Wipe outward from the eye. You can also choose to flush the eye area with lukewarm water for 15 minutes. If pain persists, seek medical advice immediately.

Avoid overexposure to essential oils by being sure there is proper ventilation. Should you feel dizzy or nauseous, get some fresh air.

Some oils on photosensitive (such as the citrus oils). Avoid sunlight and tanning beds 3-4 hours after applying these oils to your body. Should sunburn occur, apply aloe vera gel gently and sparingly to the area and avoid any addition heat to the area.

Before using a new essential oil-read all about it. Read about its properties, dosages and contraindications. Then decide if it is right for you.

Overdose

It never ceases to amaze me that the same people who believe that essential oils have healing properties to them, don't believe that they can over dose on them. You have to first remember that essential oils are 50-70 times more concentrated than herbs. It is also important to remember that while some essential oils like Ylang Ylang are sedative in small doses and that is large doses they have the opposite effect and can be simulative.

There are many conflicting reports of injury and death form essential oils but there is little scientific research that has been done on the subject. I will try to include the information that I can find on the inherent dangers of essential oils.

Too much nutmeg can make you hallucinate; oregano and cassia can cause your skin to burn. Too much rosemary essential oil can cause you to vomit, kidney irritation, muscle spasms, bleeding from the uterus, coma and even death. Pennyroyal may cause seizures, liver damage, lung damage, loss of consciousness and even death.
Eucalyptus oil can cause a burning sensation in your mouth, difficulty swallowing, seizure, drowsiness, skin irritant; can induce labor in pregnant women, shallow or rapid breathing, weak heartbeat, and swelling.

Bergamot oil can cause blurred vision, burning sensation, muscle cramping, tingling sensations and even paresthesia (altered sensations). Other essential oils that can be potentially lethal when consumed in great amounts include arnica, bitter almond, birch, camphor, mustard, parsley, peppermint, tansy, turmeric, wintergreen and wormseed.

In case of overdose, call for emergency medical assistance (911). Do not induce vomiting unless instructed by medical professional. Be sure to keep the bottle, or bottles of oils that the person has overdosed on so that you can give them to the attending medical professional.

Depending on the person and the essential oil that they have overdosed on, the person should see improvement after treatment to within days of the overdose.

Preventing Essential Oil Overdose

There are many things that you can do to prevent accidently overdosing on essential oils. Some of the same things that you can do to prevent overdosing on essential oils is the same things that you would do to prevent overdosing on other drugs.

- Follow the instructions on the bottle and your therapist.
- Always take the proper dosage.

Individual Oil and their Precaution

Essential Oil	Precautions
Basil	Avoid during pregnancy, epilepsy, photosensitive
Cassia	Photosensitive, irritates nasal membranes
Clove	Photosensitive, avoid during pregnancy
Clary Sage	Avoid during pregnancy
Coriander	May cause nausea
Eucalyptus	Avoid during pregnancy or nursing
Fennel	Avoid during pregnancy, seizures
Ginger	Skin sensitizing
Lemongrass	Skin sensitizing
Marjoram	Diminishes sex drive and function, drowsiness
Melissa	Skin sensitizing
Oregano	Skin sensitizing, avoid during pregnancy
Peppermint	Avoid with high blood pressure and homeopathy
Roman Chamomile	Avoid during pregnancy
Rosemary	Avoid during pregnancy, high blood pressure, epilepsy
Tansy	Allergic Reactions
Thyme	Avoid during pregnancy, high blood pressure. Skin sensitizing

Chapter Nine
Delivery Methods

Application of Essential Oils

Please remember that essential oils remain in the body for 20-90 minutes. Essential oils are naturally excreted from the body through exhalation, urine, and sweat. Below is a list of common uses for essential oils:

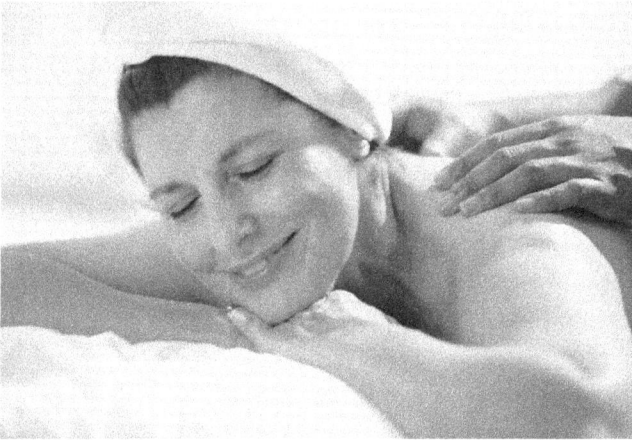

Add essential oils in a carrier oil, cream or lotion for a massage session

Topical Use: applying essential oils to the skin of the body.
Since the skin is the largest organ of the body, applying essential oil to the skin just makes sense. The skin is able to rapidly absorb the essential oil and bring it into the bloodstream. This is possible because essential oils are lipotropic (fat soluble). Also, you can massage the essential oil in a blend directly on an area of need such as massaging the abdomen for digestive problems, or massaging an area of a sore muscle, an injury, the temples for a headache, etc.
Benefits of massage include:
- Enters the blood stream within 3 minutes.
- Apply to a specific area (muscle leg cramp) or to the entire body.

- Increases lymph system
- Increases circulation system
- Prolonged use may cause phototoxicity or cause skin irritations.

Massage oil or lotions-Add essential oils to your massage oils, lotions or creams, and massage into the client, or onto affected area. Aside from massaging the area in need directly, massaging the feet will also help the client as all of the organs and organ tissues are located on the bottoms of the feet, the palms of the hand and on point on the ear. This is called *Reflexology*. You client may also be able to just apply the oil blend to the bottoms of their feet before bedtime. This will also work when a therapist is doing Acupressure. Just add 1-3 drops of oil blend to your finger (or thumb) and press and activate the acupressure point. One last thing that you can do in the massage session with your oils is called *layering*. In layering, you may use one oil blend on the body first, and then when that oil blend dries, you will be able to use another oil blend over top of it. This works especially well on sore muscles where you can use rosemary to calm the muscle spasm and then peppermint to invigorate, etc.

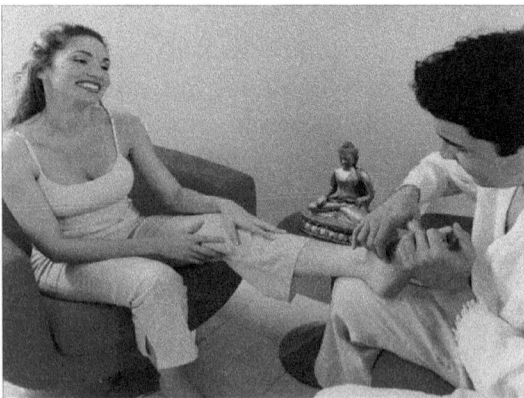

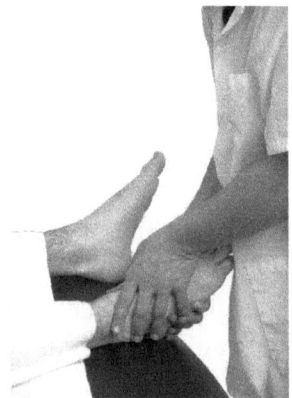

Reflexology and Foot Massages are great ways to apply oil blends

Salves-Using Golden Salve, Rescue Remedy Creams, etc., you can add essential oils to the salve to use on specific areas of the body in need.

Compresses (hot and cold)-You can a few drops of essential oil to a bowl of hot (or cold) water, soak a towel in it, wring it out, and place the towel on the area in need. A simple fever reducing recipe would be to use 4oz. of cold water, 2 drops of lemon, 1 drop of peppermint and 1 drop of lavender essential oil. Dip washcloth or towel into the water, wring it out and apply to the forehead, neck, under the armpits, or the bottoms of the feet. Leave on until towel warms (usually 5-10 minutes) and repeat.

Bath-to use essential oils in the bath, you must add the essential oil to a carrier such as bath salts, Epsom salts, carrier oils, or vodka. Be sure to remember that you while you can safely use essential oils in the bathtub for adults, great care must be taken in what oils you use for children and babies and how much is considered safe. Some oils can be toxic for children and pets so please do not use these oils. See list of precautions listed earlier in this manual.

Baths are excellent for skin problems, circulation problems, respiratory problems, stress and nervous tension, muscle aches and pains, PMS, insomnia, and more. Mix essential oils in with Epson salts or sea salts before adding to the bath (normally 5-12 drops of essential oil per bath). Prolonged use of essential oils may cause irritation.

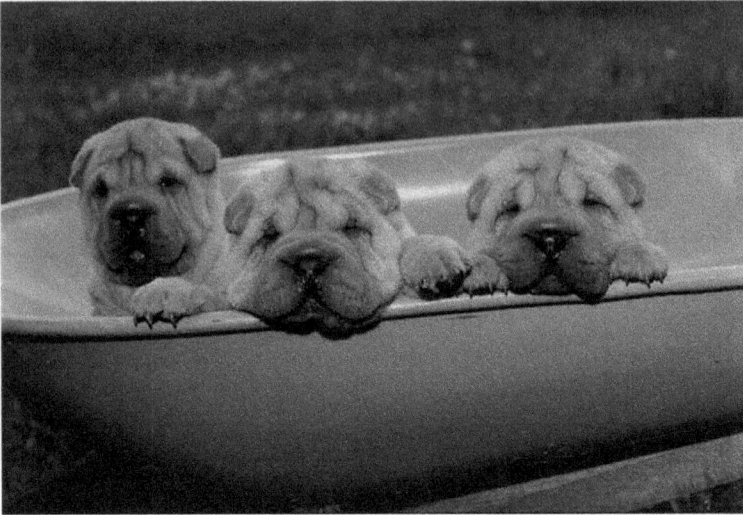

Baths-Use less essential oil in baths for children and pets

Foot Baths-Add essential oils of lavender and tea tree to a small tub of water to fight fungal infections such as athlete's feet.

Sitz Baths-Add essential oils to a small tub and sit for hemorrhoid relief.

Mouthwash-Dilute essential oil in a glass of water and vodka. Use for mouth infections, cold sores, and bad breath.

Suppository-Mix essential oils with a carrier such as Golden Salve and apply to the area. Use to help with colitis, Crohn's disease and yeast infections. Add 1-2 drops of essential oil blend to a gel capsule and insert into body cavity. Use for relief of hemorrhoids and yeast infections.

Douche-Prolonged use may cause colonic problems.

Inhalation: sniffing the essential directly from the bottle

Through inhalation we can relax or stimulate the nervous system of the body because the aromas that we breathe in affect our brains through the olfactory receptors. The receptors send impulses along olfactory nerves towards the brain where they will be interpreted and acted upon.

The sense of smell is the easiest and quickest ways to active and stimulates the limbic system of the body. Essential oil molecules enter the brain and blood via cranial nerves, nasal membranes and the alveoli in the lungs. This method is best used for respiratory issues, sinus issues and headaches. Prolonged use of concentrated oils may irritate mucus membranes and cause headaches, dizziness, and nausea.

Cotton ball, potpourri, pine cones, sachets-Just a drop or two of essential oil to items like a cotton ball and place in drawers and closets.

Room diffuser or nebulizer-Perfect for diffusing essential oils into rooms of your home or office. Also can use for the car.

Room spray, carpet deodorizer-Always a good one for when the family is sick, or to bring about a certain mood during the holidays. Covers a large area in a very quick time.

Steam (like putting a few drops of essential oils in a pot of very hot water and then placing a towel of your head and over the pot to inhale the steam.

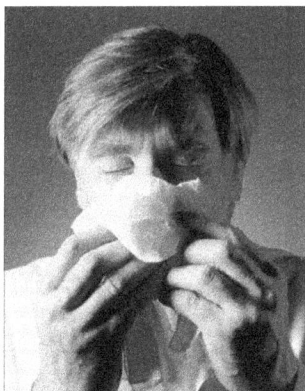

Inhalation-Inhaling essential oil that was applied to a tissue

Oral Ingestion

Because I adhere to the dictates of the National Association of Holistic Aromatherapy (NAHA), I will not give essential oils to people for oral ingestion. But that doesn't mean that all essential oils are unsafe for oral ingestion. I have included a 2013 list of food supplements and additives that the FDA feels are safe for human consumption. The FDA however, has not determined what about of consumption of any one given product is safe. This is why it is important to be under the care of a medical professional should you wish to take essential oils orally. You must also remember that unlike herbs, essential oils are highly concentrated. Most adults dosages range from 1-3 drops no more than 2-3 times a day for up to 5 days and then the body should receive a 'break' from using essential oils.

Essential oils are not recommended for ingestion by people who are pregnant, nursing, children, pets, and epileptics. Oils should be diluted before ingestion in any liquid such as water, tea, or orange juice, but not in milk as milk may make the ingredients inactive.

Some essential oils may burn the membranes of your mouth and esophagus if they are not properly diluted such as cassia, eucalyptus, oregano, ginger and cinnamon. Ingestion of oils is only for a very short period of time and prolonged use may case organ toxicity or damage.

The United States Federal Food, Drug and Cosmetic Act (the Act) has created a sheet called 'Generally Recognized as Safe (GRAS)' that includes substances that are added to food that has received approval by the FDA. The Code of Federal Regulations (CFR) is a codification of the rules of the Food and Drug Administration under Title 21. Under 21 CFR 170.30, food falls under general recognition of food safety through experience and scientific procedures. The CFR at GPO, both current and historical, can also be searched directly at: http://www.gpoaccess.gov/cfr/index.html.

More information available from the official FDA government Website and lists those essential oils, oleoresins (solvent-free), and natural extractive (including distillates) that are generally recognized as safe for their intended use at: http://www.accessdata.fda.gov/scripts/cdrh/cfdocs/cfcfr/CFRSearch.cfm?fr=182.20

Chapter Ten
Blending

Volatility

Volatility is the tendency of a substance to vaporize and is directly related to a substance's vapor pressure (pressure at which a gas phase is in balance with the condensed phase). The higher the vapor pressure, the more readily a substance vaporizes.

In Aromatherapy, essential oils that are most volatile are considered top notes. These are the oils that are the quickest to evaporate from a blend. Medium evaporating oils are called middle notes and the slowest essential oils to evaporate from a blend are called base notes. When making a blend, it is beneficial to include essential oils from the top, middle and base notes. This is accomplished by using a ratio formula of 3 drops of top notes to 2 drops of middle notes to 1 drop of base note (the 3-2-1) formula. You can also double your mixes by using 6 drops of top note to 4 drops of middle note to 2 drops of base notes (6-4-2). This type of blending isn't set in stone but it is a nice way to guarantee a more even and thorough blending, especially in perfumes.

The Properties of the Notes

- **Top Notes**-Top notes are light, fresh and evaporate quickly. It is the first scent that you are aware of in a blend and it is the first scent to leave the blend. Most of the citrus essential oils fall into this group.
- **Middle Notes**-Middle notes evaporate at a slower rate of speed and they are noted for adding stability to the top notes. The middle note is considered the body of the blend, and/or fragrance.
- **Bottom Notes**-Bottom notes are slow to evaporate. The fragrances of these essential oils are rich and full body. When used in a blend, the bottom notes take a while for the scent to emerge, but once they do, they can linger for a long time. Use essential oils from this category sparingly.

Short Chart of Essential Oils and their Notes

TOP notes	MIDDLE notes	BOTTOM notes
Basil	Bay	Balsam peru
Bergamot	Black Pepper	Cassia
Cajupet	Cardamom	Cedarwood
Clary Sage	Chamomile	Cinnamon Bark
Coriander	Cinnamon	Clove
Eucalyptus	Cypress	Frankincense
Grapefruits	Geranium	Ginger
Hyssop	Calendula	Jasmine
Lemon	Juniper	Myrrh
Lemongrass	Lavender	Neroli
Lime	Marjoram	Nutmeg
Mandarin	Melissa	Oakmoss
Myrtle	Myrtle	Patchouli
Niaouli	Palma Rosa	Rose
Orange	Pepper	Rosewood
Oregano	Peppermint	Sandalwood
Peppermint	Pine	Vervain
Petitgrain	Rosemary	Vanilla
Ravensara	Rosewood	Vetiver
Tea Tree	Spineward	Ylang Ylang
Thyme	Yarrow	

Basic Guidelines

When making the perfect blend, it is important to combine essential oils with high, middle, and base notes that complement each other. There are many ways of accomplishing this task. One way is work with a particular "family" of oils. One such family would be the citrus family; another would be the Wood family.

The citrus family of oils is notorious for being a "high" note which means that the scent of the oil disappears very quickly, making it very volatile.

The Wood family of oils tends to be more of the 'base' notes, or low notes making the scent of these oils last for a much longer time. Middle notes like Lavender and Geranium tend to make the top notes last longer, but it is the base notes that will dominate the blend if they are used in equal amounts with the middle and high notes. Here is a simple formula for you to remember when creating your next blend of essential oils:

3 – 2 – 1 to 1 ounce of carrier oil

The 3-2-1 blend stands for 3 drops of a high note, 2 drops of a middle note, and 1 drop of a base note added to 1 ounce of carrier oil. That is the basic blending formula to create the perfect blend. You can increase this basic formula to such degrees such as:

3-2-1
6-4-2
9-6-3
30-20-10

A typical recipe for making perfume is to use 25 drops of essential oil to 2 ½ ounces of carrier oil. This carrier oil can be pure grain alcohol, such as vodka, or you can just use jojoba oil. The 25 drops of essential oils that you will be using will still be based on the above 3-2-1- formula using 3 drops of top notes to every 2 drops of middle notes to 1 drop of every base note.

Fixatives such as Phthalates and Glycerin are sometimes added to the perfume to depress the evaporation rate of essential oils. Fixatives can come in either vegetable or animal while a wide range of synthetic substances are used today.

The problem with using Phthalates is that they are known to have a carcinogenic effect. Both Phthalates and Glycerin may cause or provoke allergic reactions in some people. Because of this fact, and the fact that essential oils do not evaporate very fast in the atmosphere, you may choose to leave fixatives out of your formulas, I know I do.

The important thing to remember though while you are creating your blends is KEEP NOTES! There is nothing like coming up with a wonderful finished product and then you find yourself unable to recreate it because you forgot the formula.

Another important thing to remember is that when your blend has time to sit for a while, it will change. The change may be ever so slight, but it will happen. It may even surprise and delight you. There is a lot of experimentation that goes on to create the perfect blend. With practice and patience, you will create a blend that is perfect and right for you, or your client.

Synergies

The effectiveness of any blend is dependent upon many factors. One such factor is the proportions of each essential oil used in the blend. This is vital to the effectiveness of the remedy as a whole. Some essential oils that are blended together have a mutually enhancing effect upon one another so that the whole is greater than the sum of the parts.

A good example would be the anti-inflammatory action of Chamomile which is supported by being mixed with Lavender. When blends work in harmony together, the combination is a "synergy," and every Aromatherapist wants to create a good one.

There are some things which should do in order to create a good synergy. One of these things is that you must take into account not only the symptom to be treated but also the underlying cause of the disorder, the biological, and the psychological or emotional factors involved.

This is why individual prescriptions are preferred over the mass produced "synergies" on the market today. Each blended essence is made for an individual's physical requirement, as well as, their emotional.

Essential Oils are also grouped together according to their common constituents such as camphoraceous oils containing a good percentage of cineol (members of the Mytacease group such as eucalyptus, tea tree, cajuput and myrtle.

Some essential oils such as rose, jasmine, oak moss and lavender seem to enhance just about any blend. Some combinations of essential oils have an inhibiting power over one another. You must learn the character of each essential oil before attempting blends with them.

It was a Frenchman named Piesse who instigated a new approach to classifying odors. He transformed the fragrances into corresponding notes. Together, these notes formed a balanced chord of harmony when blended together. Each essential oil is classified according to what Piesse believed to be that oils' dominant character.

Temperature

Essential oils should be stored in dark, colored glass bottles away from direct heat sources, including a window sill where the sun can reach it. Store your bottles in a cool, dark place away from children and pets.

One place where you can store your citrus essential oils, as well as some of your carrier oils, is in the refrigerator. Be sure that your refrigerator is set between 5-10 degrees Celsius.

Refrigeration is not suggested for Aniseed, Fennel, Rose Otto, and Star Anise as these oils may solidify at cold temperatures. If this happens, you can still use the essential oil once you have let it warm back up at room temperature. Essential oils are flammable so be sure not to store them near stoves, fires, candles, or other sources of heat.

Light

Essential oils should not be place where the sun can shine on it. If you place your essential oils where the sun can hit it, this will speed up the process called oxidation, which will deteriorate the overall effectiveness of the essential oil. Store all essential oils in dark colored bottles in a dark and cool storage place.

Air

Essential oils are volatile which means that they will evaporate quickly when opened. Be sure to replace the cap quickly and tightly on your bottle of essential oil when you are finished using it.

The more often a bottle is opened, the more opportunities there will be for the properties of the essential oil to dissipate which will weaken the overall effectiveness of the essential oil.

Space

Another thing to notice is the size of the bottle that you are using in relation to the amount of essential oil left in the bottle. Always try to use the small bottle possible to house the most essential oil. This is because the empty space that is created by the amount left over in the bottle will encourage and hasten the speed of oxidation in the product. If you have only 2 ounces of essential oil left over in a 4 ounce bottle, then it would be beneficial to pour the 2 ounces of essential oil in a 2 ounce bottle.

How to Detect Deterioration of an Essential Oil

There are some ways in which you can notice if the essential oil that you are using has deteriorated. Look for cloudiness, thickening, or overall smell changes.

Equipment

Use only glass containers. Wear mask and gloves. Be sure you work in an open air environment so that you do not succumb to any fumes. Be sure to take notes of everything that you create so that you make it again.

Dilution Ratio

½% dilution for cats
1% dilution for children, pets and elderly
2% dilution for whole body massage
4% dilution for concentrated ailments

Examples	Volume	1% dilution	2% dilution	3% dilution
Room spray	2 ounce bottle	10 drops	20 drops	40 drops
Massage	1 ounce bottle	5 drops	10 drops	20 drops
Face mist	.5 ounce bottle	3 drops	6 drops	12 drops

Essential Oil Dilution Chart according to Bottle Size/Carrier Oil used

Carrier	1% # drops	2% # drops	5% # drops	10% # drops	20% # drops	50% # drops
5ml	1	2	5	10	20	50
10ml	2	4	10	20	40	100
30ml	6	12	30	60	120	300
50ml	10	20	50	100	200	500
100ml	20	40	100	200	400	1000

Please note that anything more than 2% dilution should only be done by a trained Aromatherapist as they must be able to monitor their client carefully.

Measurements (approximation):
1 ml...20-30 drops,
5 ml...1 tsp. or 1/6 ounce, 100 drops
10 ml...2 teaspoons or 1/3 ounces
15 ml...1 tablespoon or ½ ounce
30 ml...1 ounce or 2 tablespoons
60 ml...2 ounces or ¼ cup
120 mil...4 ounces or ½ cup
75 drops.......1 teaspoon
450 drops.....1 ounce
8 grams.........1 ounce
28.5 grams...1 ounce
3 teaspoons=1 tablespoon
16 tablespoons=1 cup
1 cup=8 ounces
2 cups=1 pint
4 cups=1 quart
4 quarts=1 gallon

Worksheet to Make your Blend

1. Begin with your bottle (choose dark or colored glass).
2. Decide the purpose of your blend and write it down (i.e. relaxing, healing, chest rub, aching muscle massage lotion, etc.)
3. Make a list of the essential oils that will help with the purpose of the blend. Give priority to the list of essentials oils
4. Make a list of all of the carrier oils that will help with the purpose of the blend. Give priority to the list of carrier oils
5. Cross out all essential oils that will be contraindicated.
6. Cross out all carrier oils that will be contraindicated.
7. Narrow down your choice of essential & carrier oils to five or less.
8. Decide how much of a blend/bottles, you are going to make.

NOTE: I only use the 3-2-1- blending method if I am making products for resale.

Chapter Eleven
Carrier Oils

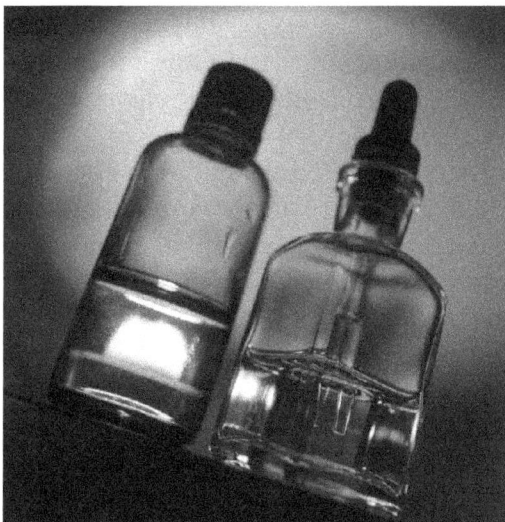

When selecting your carrier oils there are many things to take into account, how you will ultimately use the blend. Whatever carrier oil you use, remember that the properties of that oil will be added to your end product. For healing salves, I prefer to use olive oil to which I add Vitamin E to prolong the shelf life of the product. For creams and lotions, I am careful to discover the particular needs of the person who will be using the product. I take into consideration any and all contraindications that the user may have. For instance, if a person suffers from hay fever, I would not make them a product using Calendula carrier oils. Or, if a person was allergic to peanuts, I wouldn't use oil that contained nuts such as Sweet Almond, Hazelnut, Macadamia Nut, or Peanut Oil.

Following is a short list of carrier oils and their properties. There are many carrier oils to choose from but I have tried to list some of the most popular one below. For more information, please do more research by reading some of the fine books I have listed in the Reference section of this booklet. For massage purposes, use cold-pressed oils as they are absorbed more easily into the skin. Some good chooses would be sweet almond, sunflower, grape seed and coconut oil.

List of some Carrier Oils

Aloe Vera-(Aloe Vera)-Great for use in wound healing, sunburns, skin
  that is hot to the touch. Very cooling and refreshing.

Apricot Kernel-(Armeniaca vulgaris, Prunis armeniaca) - good facial
  oil; Vitamins A, B. Aids in healing/rejuvenating skin cells. Use on
  mature, dry and damaged skin.

Avocado-(Persea Americana, Persea gratissima) - good for dry, flaky,
  and aging skin types; rich and heavy with minor sunscreen effects.
  Expensive. Great to combine with other carrier oils in a blend. Oil
  is thick, rich and green in color. High in Vitamins A, D, E,
  lecithin and potassium (among others). Use on chapped hands,
  rashes, chaffing and even on babies for cradle cap.

Baking Soda-(sodium bicarbonate)-Used to absorb perspiration and
  odors, cleans carpets.

Calendula oil-(Calendula officinalis) - good as a body oil; speeds up
  healing/moisturizing for dry/damaged skin.

Carrot oil- (*Daucus carota L. var. Chantenay, fam. Apiaceae
  (Umbelliferae)*-Rich in Vitamin A and bet-carotene. Carrot oil
  can be used in conjunction with any skin healing essential oil
  blend. Use for liver disorders, gallbladder problems, hepatitis,
  colitis, ulcers and abscesses. Use for hair and skin tone, scars and
  acne. Great in anti-aging skin care products.

Castor oil (Ricinus communis L) - good for sealing in moisture; a
  heavy oil that seals and protects.

Coconut Oil (Unfractionated)-Use to moisturize and refresh skin.
  Easily absorbed into the skin.

Colloidal Silver-pure silver suspended in distilled water.

Epson Salt-(magnesium sulfate). Use to detoxify the skin, relieve sore
  muscles.

Evening Primrose – (Oemothera biennis)-antioxidant. Often added to
  other Carrier Oils to prolong shelf life.

Grapeseed-(Vitis vinifera) - good as a massage oil and facial oil; very
  light, penetrates the skin quickly. Slightly astringent (use for acne,
  oily skin), facial toner, cellulite, skin tightening. Relatively
  inexpensive.

Hazelnut oil – (Corylus avellana) - good for facials; loaded with vitamins, minerals and proteins. High Vitamins A, B, E and linoleic acid. Great skin absorption.

Hemp-(Canabis sativa)-reduces roughness and irritation. Good for cracked hands and feet.

Jojoba oil-(Simmondsia sinensis, Buxux sinensis) - very dry/oily skin; often added to other Carrier Oils to prolong their shelf life. Not an oil as such but a liquid was, makes this oil more stable than other oils and the first choice in making blends for resale (since they can have a shelf life of 10 or more years). Use for skin conditions such as rashes, psoriasis and eczema.

Macadamia-(Macadamia tenuifolia)-use for eczema, dry chapped skin, psoriasis and burns. This oil is rich in palmitoleic acid which is great for delaying the onset of skin and cell damage.

Olive oil-(Olea europaea) - "extra virgin" has the highest amount of vitamins and minerals. Great to use in homemade soaps and shampoos. Little thick so you can mix with other oils.

Safflower Oil-(Carthamus tinctorius Flos.) - good for softening the kin; it's a light-to-medium weight oil.

Shea Butter-vitellaria paradoza-Thick wax from Shea nuts for wound and skin healing.

St. John's Wort-(*Hypericum perforatum)*-also known as Hypericum oil is used for soft tissue injuries. Good to use for neuralgia, shingles, RA, and other ailments that result in pain in the nerve endings.

Sunflower oil-(Helianthus annuus) - good for massage, body lotions, and body oils; rich in Vitamin E. Cold-pressed sunflower oil is best to use as it contains essential fatty acids beneficial for skin healing treatments.

Sweet Almond-(prunus amygdalus, P. dulcis)-Great to use on dry and itchy skin. Also good for skin that is inflamed. Works well in massage oil blends. Sweet and lightweight.

Vitamin E oil - good for prolonging the shelf life of other Carrier Oils; very thick; Use in 10% dilution to preserve a blend. Antioxidant properties; heals scar tissue and rejuvenates skin cellular activity. Great for mature skin, scar tissue or stretch marks. Great source of unsaturated fatty acids and Vitamins A and E.

Wheatgerm oil-(Triticum saivum) - good for healing scars, burns and stretch marks; Vitamins A, D, and E

Please remember that a carrier oil can be anything that you put essential oils into which includes bath water, honey, dead sea salts, lotions, creams, gels, etc.

Chapter Twelve
Essential Oils

Aromatherapy and Your Pet
Just like in humans, aromatherapy can help canines physically, mentally and emotionally. Dogs suffer from some of the same situations that humans do such as separation anxiety, stress, irritability, and pain.

Since dogs cannot communicate with humans with language, they can only act out by barking, snapping, clawing, hiding, etc. It is up to their human counterparts to try to figure out what is going on with their pet, or to allow a vet to intervene.

When a pet is barking, try to look for the reason behind the barking. Are they being overstimulated, are they afraid, or stressed? If you want to calm down a pet, look for essential oils such as lavender or chamomile.Or if your dog is anxious, stressed or full of tension, the same calming essential oils of lavender or chamomile may help. Some other calming essential oils that are safe to use for your pet is listed below:

Calming Your Dog with Essential Oils

Essential Oil	Use to
Cardamon	Nausea, Appetite, Weight Loss, Heartburn, Anti-bacterial
Cedar	Flea Control
Chamomile (both)	Anti-inflammatory, Nausea, Skin issues
Clary Sage	Calms the Nerves
Eucalyptus	Controls Fleas and Ticks, Parasites, Soothes Insect Bites and Stings and Skin Rashes
Frankincense	Anti-bacterial, wound healing
Lavender	Inflammation, Bacteria, Burns, Cuts, Bruises, Motion Sickness, Anxiety, Stress, Tension
Lemongrass	Repels Fleas and Ticks, Aids in Skin Conditions
Peppermint	Treats arthritis, strains and sprains
Spearmint	Nausea, Diarrhea
Thyme	Pain relief, Infections, Arthritis, or Rheumatism. Aids in skin issues

Essential Oils to <u>Avoid</u> Using Around Dogs
    Although there is still some discussion about what is truly safe for your pet, I would absolutely avoid diffusing the following oils. Some of these oils may be safe in a very small dilution for a short period of time but why take the chance when there are so many other oils that you can use:

- Citrus oils such as lemon, orange, or tangerine
- Tea tree
- Ylang ylang
- Cinnamon
- Pennyroyal
- Pine
- Sweet Birch
- Juniper
- Nutmeg
- Wintergreen

Essential Oils <u>Safe</u> to Use with Dogs
- Angelica Root Angelica archangelica
- Basil (linalool chemotype) Ocimum basilicum ct. linalool
- Bergamot Citrus bergamia, Citrus aurantium subspecies bergamia
- Black Pepper Piper nigrum
- Cajeput Melaleuca cajuputi
- Caraway Carum carvi
- Cardamom Elatteria cardamomum
- Carrot Seed Daucus carota, Daucus carota subspecies sativa
- Cedarwood (Atlas) Cedrus atlantica
- Chamomile (German) Matricaria chamomilla, Matricaria recutita, Chamomilla recutita
- Chamomile (Roman) Anthemis nobilis, Chamaemelum nobile
- Cistus Cistus ladanifer, Cistus ladaniferus
- Citronella Cymbopogon winterianus, Cymbopogon nardus
- Coriander Coriandrum sativum
- Cypress Cupressus sempervirens
- Elemi Canarium luzonicum, Canarium vulgare

- Eucalyptus Eucalyptus radiata (this is the species specified, but the other species have the same safety issues)
- Fennel (Sweet) Foeniculum vulgare
- Frankincense Boswellia carterii (this is the species specified, but the other species have the same safety issues, with the exception of Boswellia papyfera which is not recommended to use during pregnancy for humans)
- Geranium Pelargonium graveolens, Pelargonium x asperum
- Ginger Zingiber officinale
- Helichrysum Helichrysum italicum and Helichrysum splendidum
- Lavender Lavender angustifolia, Lavender officinalis
- Lemongrass Cymbopogon flexuosus, Andropogon flexuosus, Cymbopogon citratus, Andropogon citratus
- Mandarin Citrus reticulata, Citrus nobilis
- Marjoram (Sweet) Origanum marjorana, Marjorana hortensis, Origanum dubium
- Melissa Melissa officinalis
- Myrrh Commiphora myrrha, Commiphora molmol
- Neroli Citrus x aurantium
- Niaouli Melaleuca quinquinervia
- Opopanax Commiphora erythraea, Commiphora guidottii
- Palmarosa Cymbopogon martinii, Andropogon martinii var martinii, Cymbopogon martinii var motia
- Patchouli Pogostemon cablin, Pogostemon patchouly
- Peppermint Mentha piperita
- Petitgrain Citrus aurantium
- Plai Zingiber cassumunar, Zingiber montanum, Amomum montanum, Zingiber purpureum
- Rosalina Melaleuca ericifolia
- Rose (Bulgarian, Damask) Rosa damascena (this is the species specified, but it's actually the Rose which needs the most dilution, so it stands to reason the other Rose species are also safe)
- Rosemary Rosmarinus officinalis
- Sandalwood Santalum spicatum, Santalum album (this essential oil was not listed in either book below, but was verified to be safe by Kelly who runs the EO animal group)

- Spearmint Mentha spicata, Mentha cardiaca, Mentha crispa, Mentha viridis
- Spikenard Nardostachys grandiflora
- Tangerine Citrus reticulata, Citrus nobilis, Citrus tangerine
- Thyme (linalool chemotype) Thymus vulgaris ct. linalool
- Valerian Valeriana officinalis
- Vanilla Vanilla planifolia, Vanilla fragrans, Vanilla tahitensis
- Vetiver Vetiveria zizanoides, Andropogon muricatus, Andropogon zizanoides, Chrysopogon zizanoides, Phalaris zizanoides
- Yarrow Achillea millefolium
- Ylang Ylang Cananga odorata, Cananga odorata genuina

Here are some Oil Profiles

Essential Oil #1: Helichrysum, known as *Everlasting Essential Oil* or *Immortelle*.
Botanical Name: Helichrysum italicum (everlasting or immortelle)
Aromatic Scent: Warm, earthy and bittersweet
Plant Part: Flowering Tops of Plant
Extraction Method: Steam Distilled
Country of Origin: Croatia
Color: Pale yellow
Viscosity: Thin
Distillation Method: Steam-distillation
Blends well with: Chamomile, Lavender, Clary Sage, and Rose.

On the Emotional Level: Use this oil to open the Heart Chakra, clear old emotional wounds, let go of grudges and resentments, learn to forgive others and to be forgiven. Use to unblock/regulate energy in the body, release of Qi (Chi), restore compassion.

On the Physical Level: Use this oil for healing the skin, scars and wounds. Release muscle knots, anti-inflammatory, chelation (use on soles of feet to remove metals from the body), tissue rejuvenation, burn healing, reduce swelling, back and neck pain reduction, reduce surgical scarring, use on arthritic conditions, dissipates free radicals, analgesic, supports liver function, use on areas for numbness and tingling. May also help those with hearing loss/damage or suffer from tinnitus (just place a drop of essential oil on cotton ball and place it in the ear while sleeping each night for two weeks).

Caution: For external use only. Do not use directly on skin, dilute in a carrier oil. If skin sensitivity occurs, discontinue use. If you are pregnant, nursing or taking any medications, consult your doctor before use.

Essential Oil #5: Sweet Thyme
Botanical Name: Thymus vulgaris ct. linalol
Aromatic Scent: Fresh herbaceous aroma
Plant Part: leaves
Oil Characteristics: Antiseptic, antiviral, diuretic, carminative, antispasmodic, expectorant, antibacterial, disinfectant, stimulant, astringent, insecticide, febrifuge and antiparasitic.
Extraction Method: Steam Distilled
Country of Origin: n/a
Color: Clear to pale yellow
Viscosity: Thin to medium
Blends well with: All citrus oils, chamomile, lavender, frankincense, geranium, eucalyptus, myrrh, rosewood, sandalwood, vetiver, rosemary, oregano and pine
On the Emotional Level: Use for mental exhaustion.
On the Physical Level: Insect repellant
Mouthwash and gargle for sore throats or gum problems
Colds, flu, whooping cough, bronchitis, respiratory catarrh. Clears excess mucus from lungs. Use for asthma.
Digestive aid, flatulence. Use for gout and intestinal parasites. Gastritis.
Epilepsy
Kills bacteria and airborne viruses.
Stimulates circulation.

Caution: too much can contraindicated for people with high blood pressure.

Essential Oil 12#: Fennel
Botanical Name: Foeniculum vulgare
Aromatic Scent: Sweet and slightly spicy
Plant Part: Seeds
Oil Characteristics: antiseptic, antispasmodic, carminative, depurative, diuretic, emmenagogue, expectorant, galactagogue, laxative, stimulant, stomachic, splenic, tonic and vermifuge.
Extraction Method: Steam Distilled
Country of Origin: Mediterranean
Color: Clear to pale yellow
Viscosity: Thin
Blends well with: Geranium, lavender, rose and sandalwood
On the Emotional Level: Calms the nerves
On the Physical Level: Good digestive aid. Stimulates the release of bile from the liver
   Use to detoxify the body
   Use for gout, rheumatoid arthritis, cellulite. Use for kidney stones
   Use as a tonic to strengthen after a bout of illness of exhaustion
   In Europe, given to babies in a dilution of 0.5% in massage for colic
   Use for PMS and menopausal problem (has estrogenic action)
   Decreases appetite, aids weight loss, increases stamina
   Use to promote lactation and urination

Caution: Avoid if you have tumors or cysts that are estrogen based.

Essential Oil #13: Basil, Exotic
Botanical Name: Ocimum basilicum
Country Grown: India
Viscosity: Thin like water
Actions: Aphrodisiac, Insect Repellent, Uplifting, Anti-Depressant, Soothing, Antiseptic, Stomachic, Digestive, Tonic
Characteristics: Faint Licorice scent. Sharp and warm.
Method: Steam Distillation
Note: Top
Physical Uses: Energizing, elevating and anti-depressive
        Use with children who have ADD and ADHD to help them focus
        Clears a fogged head
        Helps the Mind to focus
        Helps with memory
        Use when working on creative/intellectual tasks (like studying for test)
        Bronchitis
        Headaches and Migraines
Emotional Uses: Anti-Depressive, energizing, elevating
Blends well with: Eucalyptus, Geranium, Tea Tree, Lavender, Bergamot
Contraindications: Avoid during pregnancy. Could irritate or sensitize delicate skin. May irritate eyes. If irritation persists, call a physician, remove contact lenses and flush eyes with cool water for 15-20 minutes. Remove contaminated clothing and wash skin with mild soap and water.

Essential Oil #14: Sweet Marjoram
Botanical Name: Origana marjorana
Country: Hungary using the wildcrafted method
Viscosity: Thin like water
Note: Middle
Actions: Anaphrodisiac (reduces sexual desire) Respiratory problems,
Warming, Tonic, Soothing, Relaxant, Antiseptic, digestive.
Analgesic, anti-oxidant, antiviral, bactericidal, carminative,
cephalic, cordial, diaphoretic, digestive, diuretic, emmenagogue,
expectorant, fungicidal, hypotensive, laxative, nervine, sedative,
stomachic, tonic, vulnerary
Characteristics: Warm and spicy
Method: Steam Distillation from flowers
Physical Uses: Use in a compress to relieve stomach and digestive
problems
Use for insomnia sufferers
Use to reduce muscle tension
Use to reduce inflammation and spasms
Use for respiratory problems, asthma, colds and flu
Use to help balance blood pressure
Use to help relieve Arthritis and Rheumatism
Emotional Uses: Eases feelings of loneliness and rejection
Blends well with: Peppermint, Eucalyptus, Clary Sage, Lavender,
Roman Chamomile, Bergamot, Rosemary
Contraindications: Do not use during pregnancy

Use in soaps, detergents, cosmetic and perfumes

Essential Oil: #16: German Chamomile
Botanical Name: Matricaria chamomilla
   Also known as: **Wild Camomile, True Camomile, Scented Mayweed**
Country: Switzerland, Germany
Viscosity: Medium
Actions: Analgesic, Anti-anemic, Antineuralgic, Antiphlogistic, Antiseptic, Antispasmodic, Bactericide, Carminative, Cholagogue, Cicatrizant, Digestive, Emmenogogue, Febrifuge, Hepatic, Hypnotic, Nerve Sedative, Stomachic, Sudorific, Tonic, Vermifuge, Vulnerary
Characteristics: Oil has a warm and herbaceous scent.
Method: Steam-distillation
Physical Uses: Use as a tea for children who suffer from cramps and/or stomach aches.
   Helps with flatulence, gas, diarrhea, menstrual cramps, abdominal discomfort,
   Inflammation of the testicles, increases perspiration
   Use as a compress for inflamed eyes and conjunctivitis (soothing), hemorrhoids
   Use as a compress for skin eruptions (soothing) for itching, wounds
   Use in a tea to gargle for toothache
   Use as a face wash for healthier skin and as a hair conditioner (blonde hair) for a healthy shine.
   Fever, neuralgia, rheumatic pains
Emotional Uses: Soothing and sedative
Blends well with: Bergamot, clary sage, rose geranium and lavender.
Contraindications: Allergy to ragweed

Essential Oil: #20: Black Pepper
Botanical Name: Piper nigrum
Country: India, Malaysia, Madagascar, (Singapore) China and
     Indonesia
Viscosity: Thin
Actions: analgesic, antiseptic, antispasmodic, antitoxic, aphrodisiac,
     diaphoretic, digestive, diuretic, febrifuge, laxative, rubefacient
     and tonic
Characteristics: Warm and spicy with a color from light amber to
     yellow-green.
Method: Steam-distillation
Note: Middle
Physical Uses: Increases warmth in body and mind, boosts the immune
     system (tones the spleen), and tones the digestive system.
     Stimulates the digestive system, the kidneys and circulation to
          the skin
     Relieves sore muscles and joints, exhaustion, fevers
     Pain relief, rheumatism, colds and flu, muscular aches, bruising,
          arthritis
     Stimulates appetite and encourages peristalsis, increases the flow
          of saliva
     Tones the colon muscles
Emotional Uses: Relieve coldness
Blends well with: Bergamot, clary sage, clove, coriander, fennel,
     frankincense, geranium, ginger, grapefruit, lavender, juniper,
     lemon, lime, mandarin, sage and ylang ylang.

Contraindications: May cause skin irritation. Avoid in pregnancy.
     May over-stimulate the kidneys.

Essential Oil: #21: Citronella
Botanical Name: Cymbopogon nardus (also known as Andropogon nardus)
Country: Sri Lanka and Java
Viscosity: Medium
Actions: Antiseptic, bactericidal, deodorant, diaphoretic, insecticide, parasitic, tonic and stimulant
Characteristics: Slightly sweet and lemony smell
Method: Steam-distillation
Note: Top/Middle
Physical Uses: Insect repellant, room freshener, candle wax, deordorizing
  Use in skin care products to soften skin, balance oily skin and sweaty feet
  Used in deodorants, perfumes, skin lotions and soaps
  General toning effect on the body, balances perspiration, reduces fever
  Use to fight against colds, flu and minor infections (including intestinal parasites)
Emotional Uses: Clears the mind
Blends well with: Bergamot, geranium, lemon, orange, lavender and pine
Contraindications: Avoid if you have estrogen fed tumors or cysts. May cause dermatitis. May irriate sensitive skin.

Essential Oil: #23: Dill
Botanical Name: Anethum sowa - also known as Indian Dill
Country: South West Asia
Viscosity: Thin
Actions: Antispasmodic, carminative, digestive, disinfectant, galactagogue, sedative, stomachic and sudorific.
Characteristics: Pale yellow with grassy smell
Method: Steam-distillation
Note: Top/Middle
Physical Uses: Assists with digestion (eases constipation and flatulence), hiccups,
Promotes wound healing, helps with excess sweating due to nervous tension
Calms headaches, stimulates milk flow in nursing mothers,
Emotional Uses: Combats feelings of being overwhelmed in times of crisis and/or trauma. Eases the mind.
Blends well with: Bergamot, caraway, nutmeg, all citrus oils.
Contraindications: Avoid during pregnancy

Essential Oil: #24: Thyme

Botanical Name: Thymus vulgaris (also known as Thymus aestivus, T. ilerdensis and T. velantianus)

Country Grown: Southern Europe, the Mediterranean, Asia Minor, and Central Asia, and cultivated in North America

Viscosity: Thin/Medium

Actions: Antirheumatic, antiseptic, antispasmodic, bactericidal, bechic, cardiac, carminative, cicatrisant, diuretic, emmenagogue, expectorant, hypertensive, insecticide, stimulant, tonic and vermifuge.

Characteristics: Sweet herby smell and reddish-brown to amber in color.

Method: Steam-distillation

Note: Middle

Physical Uses: Helps with memory, concentration and focus.
Used in incense in Greek temples. Used in Egyptian embalming process.
Stimulates the lung and bronchia, helps with bronchitis, coughs, colds, asthma, etc
Warms arthritis, rheumatism, sciatica and gout, poor circulation
Muscular aches and pains, sprains; Helps cellulite and obesity and edema.
Strengthens the nerves, fights feelings of exhaustion and depression
Tones the lung against colds, flu, coughs, asthma, laryngitis, sinusitis, sore throats and tonsillitis, etc. Boosts the immune system. Helps against chills and infectious diseases. As a urinary antiseptic it helps cystitis and urethritis.

Emotional Uses: Combats depression and feelings of exhaustion.

Blends well with: Bergamot, grapefruit, lemon, lavender, rosemary and pine

Contraindications: May cause skin irritation. Avoid during pregnancy. Avoid if you have high blood pressure. Do not use in skin care products.

Chapter Thirteen
Professional Issues

Documentation

Documentation is the process of collecting written information from your client regarding their past and current health history and care. This is also called the Client In-take Form or the Consent Form. This document will create a picture of your client's overall health, as well as, a basis for the assessment session and future treatment plant. This is the beginning of collecting information for your client's records. If the client has other documentations, such as x-rays, list of prescription medicines they are taking, etc., I will make copies of them and place them in the client's files.

This information should all be place in your client's folder. It is important to keep proper documentation on your client, not only for liability issue should they arise, but also because of the Health Insurance Portability and Accountability Act (HIPAA). This Act makes it possible for your client to share their information between your office and other health care providers. This is the way professionals should handle their clients. I can't tell you how many times I went to a massage therapist and didn't fill out any paperwork at all. They have no idea what my contraindications are or any of my medical history at all. Either they don't care, or they haven't been trained properly to handle any issues, or they are just cheating the IRS out of money which they don't plan on claiming on their income tax.

For the therapist, the documentation process helps them to choose what modality they will use, what areas to avoid or focus on, and to make judgments on amount of pressure to use depending upon the current health and needs of the client. The information that you collect in the above process is also legal evidence that may protect you or your business from being sued. Documentation established professional accountability and decreases the liability risk by the information that your client shared with you and it supports your chosen course of treatment.

In addition to diminishing your liability risk, documentation also helps in payment reimbursement, future research gathering data, improves quality of care, and demonstrates that the therapist followed accepted standards of care.

This is why everything should be documented. I even document every bruise, and their location, when a client comes in before I start the treatment protocols. Because you will forget a lot of information after a client leaves and you don't see them for another week or month, or perhaps even longer. I once had a client come back to me stating that one of my therapists had given her a bruise during treatment. I pulled her file and was happy to see that the therapist was efficient enough to have documented the finding of the bruise before she began the treatment session and had asked the client about it. Then the client remembered having talked with the therapist about it. See, this is how documentation can protect you and your reputation.

The Treatment Plan

The treatment plan is a course of action that outlines the steps that you, the therapist, will do to help your client achieve their health care goals. This plan can shift and change as your client improves, or worsens, as the case may be. But this too should be in writing and placed in your client's folder.

Another form of documentation, especially for massage therapists and body workers, is called SOAP notes. Soap notes are what I use in every treatment session and it has you documenting the 'subjective' 'objective' 'assessment' and 'plan.' How this is done is when a client comes in for treatment, you will write down everything that your client says is wrong with them (the reason that they come in to seek treatment) under the S-Subjective section. The next section deals with the O-Objective and this is where the therapist will write down their visual and palpatory findings, and results of any tests that they are having the client to (such as range of motion results).

The A-Assessment section deals with the physician's diagnosis (if there is one) and everything that the therapist did in the session. The last section is the P-Plan section which contains the treatment plan.

In this section, the therapist will write done the type, duration and result of the modalities and techniques used for the current issue, as well as, for future visits.

There are other variations to the SOAP notes. One other is the APIE which stands for Assessment, Plan, Implementation and Evaluation. There isn't one form of documentation that is better than the other one. You will have to choose which one makes the best sense to you and which one you will not have trouble in completing each client session. Remember, filling out these forms is as much for your benefit as they are for your client's.

Be sure to place the SOAP notes in your client's charts at the end of each session. I always review the client's charts, and my notes, when the client returns for a follow-up session. I do this well before the client arrives at my office. My first question to them would be to see how they responded to their last treatment session. I will note anything that they say to me in the current weeks' note.

Client Records

Client records are considered the property of the owners at the facility where the client has come for treatment, no matter the therapist was who did the work on them. If the therapist, who does the work on the client, also owns the facility, then the records belong to the therapist.

All records are required to be kept in a locked file cabinet for at least 4-7 years (depending on what state you live in) from the date of the last client session. Be aware that you may be subpoenaed by a court of law to give testimony about your client, especially if they have been in an auto accident. Your records will then be used to paint a picture of your client's health care needs and what you have done for your client. So be sure that you keep your writing professional as many professions will be looking at them. I already know of three cases where this has happened and only two of them kept any notes at all.

Scope of Practice

In order to legally practice aromatherapy in your state, you must check with local rules and laws regarding such practice. Since I live in the State of Florida, I can only tell you what the laws are in regards to practicing Aromatherapy at this time. In the State of Florida there are currently NO laws that prohibit a person from using, promoting, selling, and otherwise teaching aromatherapy classes. The laws as they relate to having a business DO count though.

Laws as they govern business practices are the following: A business license with your city or county municipalities to operate a business (which means you must operate a business legally in an area specifically designed for the operation of said business), apply for sales tax number is applicable, follow proper advertising procedures (no wild claims or promises), etc. More of these issues are covered in detail in the Aromatherapy Business Plan course. There are also labeling laws that can affect the sale of your product and we will be discussing these a little later in the course.

Additional Education and Resources

There are always new findings in the Aromatherapy industry and it would be extremely professional of you to keep abreast of new research findings. There are classes and workshops help all over the country, as well as new books being published.

For up-to-date information you can check the website at www.NAHA.org or www.CropWatch.org. As more information comes in, I will also try to post them on my website at www.AromaCareBooks.com

Quality of Essential Oils

Currently, there are no quality standards or governmental issues to authenticate or judge the quality or performance of essential oils. There is not one set of standards in the United States on which to base the quality of essential oils on. The flowers and plants that are used to make essential oils are grown all over the world. Each grower and manufacturer has their own set of standards, integrity and practices on how they grow, harvest and create the final product-the essential oil.

As a consumer of essential oils, it will be up to you to assess the quality of the oils that you purchase and use. But there are some things that you can do that will help you to ascertain what a good product would be. There are some regulating and certifying organizations that may help.

One such regulating board is the Federal Food and Drug Administration (FDA). Under this governmental organization we have the Federal Food, Drug and Cosmetic Act (FDCA) and the Dietary Supplement Health and Education Act (DSHEA). The FDA is responsible for regulating food safety, labeling, dietary supplements, cosmetics, food allergens, food preparations and foodborne illness, infant formula, nutrition, production information, recalls and consumer advisories, education resource library, and more. The FDA also offers specific information for people with cancer, HIV/AIDS, pregnant, older adults, diabetics, transplant recipients, infants and toddlers.

The FDA has placed essential oils under either the cosmetic or drug category depending on how the essential oil is intended for use. These two categories are regulated very differently.

As a drug, the FDA will have more regulations on the safety and quality of the essential oil and consumers would need a prescription to purchase them (which is why most essential oils are not considered drugs). An essential oil will generally fall under the cosmetic category along with foods and flavoring agents.

The Federal Trade Commission regulates claims made in advertising but not product labeling. The Consumer Product Safety Commission is responsible for room fragrance systems, odor control systems, deodorizers, etc.

The FDA does NOT define what it means when a product says that it is 'hypoallergenic.' The FDA also does not define what the words 'organic' or 'natural' mean. That is why you can see labels stating that a chicken is organic or natural (because the chicken itself is both of these in loose terminologies) but it could have been raised in a pen and given growth hormones. So it is up to the consumer to research the products that they are purchasing and using.

Should you experience a bad reaction to a cosmetic (or essential oil), then you should do the following:
Stop using the product immediately

Call your primary care physician to find ways to care for your reaction. Report serious problems to the FDA by calling 1-800-332-1088 or file online at www.fda.gov/medwatch/report.htm.

Understanding Cosmetic Labels
- Read list of ingredients to see if it contains something that you are allergic to. (If a product doesn't list its ingredients-I don't buy it.)
- Read the warnings on the label.
- Read the tips (if they exist) on the label.
- Hypoallergenic does not mean that it won't cause allergic reactions.
- Words like 'organic' or 'natural' does not mean that the product is safe.
- Check the expiration date of the products that you are going to use. (If a product doesn't list an expiration date-then I don't buy it).

The Law and Labeling

If you market your cosmetics to consumers on a retail basis (stores, online, home parties, conferences, door-to-door, etc.), then they must meet ingredient labeling requirements under the Fair Packaging and Labeling Act (FPLA). We will discuss more on labeling later in the course.

According to the FDA's regulation of cosmetics under the Federal Food, Drug and Cosmetic Act, cosmetics must not be adulterated or misbranded and it must be safe for consumers under labeled or customary conditions of use. Any color additives to the product must be approved for intended use. Packaging and labeling must not be deceptive, and must meet ingredient labeling requirements.

Outside of color additives, the law does not require cosmetic products and ingredients to be approved by the FDA before they go to market. It is your responsibility to ensure that your products are in compliance with all laws and regulations that apply to them, including proper labeling and product safety.

Cosmetics include products that cleanse the body, change a person' appearance and make a person more attractive. Products in this category include makeup, lipsticks, nail care products, perfumes, colognes, deodorants, hair dyes, shampoos, makeup removers, moisturizers, etc. The FDCA defines cosmetics by their 'intended use.' Cosmetics include products that are created to be poured, rubbed, sprinkled, or sprayed on the human body. These products are made for cleansing, altering the appearance, beautifying or promoting attractiveness.

If a product is intended to affect the way a person's body work, or is used to treat or prevent a disease, then this product is considered a drug under FDA rules and regulations. The FDA will look at the claims that the company is making with their product to make a ruling. Some products can be both a cosmetic and a drug. Be aware that if you plan on marketing your product as a drug then it must have pre-approval by the FDA.

The FDA encourages all domestic and foreign cosmetic firms to register their product formulations with the Voluntary Cosmetic Registration Program (VCRP).

This is a voluntary request and submitting your product information to VCRP does not indicate FDA approval. Only cosmetics currently available on the market in this country are eligible for registration on VCRP. The Bioterrorism Act of 2002 requires that all cosmetic ingredients that are also classified as a food product must meet certain requirements to registration.

For those who are making cosmetic products in their own home, it is completely legal to do so as far as the FDA is concerned. You will have to check with you state and local zoning laws before you set up shop in your basement. As long as the environment that you are working in will not adulterate your products (like dog hair getting into the mix, etc.), then you should be fine. The Good Manufacturing Practice (GMP) is a list of factors that an FDA investigator would look at during an inspection. This list will help you to understand how products and ingredients should be handled in order to insure their safety.

List of possible contamination (adulterated).
- Microbial contamination
- Color additive misuse
- Using prohibitive ingredients
- Using restricted ingredients
- Using packaging whose composition may injure health
- Unwanted substances showing up in the product (hair, nail, etc.)

Safety Data

You can use safety data that is published on products from the manufacturer, wholesaler or that is published in scientific journals such as on PubMed, TOXNET and on governmental websites. The Cosmetic Ingredient Review (CPR) is a website that contains information on the safety of cosmetic ingredients. It is operated by industry-funded panel of scientific and medical experts.

Does Aromatherapy fall under cosmetics or drugs?

When fragrance products are advertised as helping to improve a person's well-being in a variety of ways such as 'strengthening the immune system,' then these fragrance products are known as *behavioral fragrances* or *aromatherapy* products. While perfumes are considered as 'cosmetics' by the FDA, claims that a scent helps insomnia, helps in smoking cessation, or prevent a condition or disease, will have

The FDCA defines a drug by its intended use in the diagnosis, cure, treatment, mitigation or prevention of disease. That will affect the structure or function of the body of a human being or animal.

But what happens when a product is both a drug and a cosmetic such as an antidandruff shampoo that both cleanses the hair and treats dandruff? These products include deodorants, antiperspirants, moisturizers, toothpaste that contains fluoride, etc., must comply with the requirement from both cosmetics and drugs.

Cosmetic products and their ingredients (except for color additives), do not require FDA approval. Drugs do require FDA approval before they can be sold to the public.

In order to start the process of getting FDA approval you will have to fill out the New Drug Application (NDA) where you will confirm to a "monograph" (rules) for a particular drug category.

Soap

Soap is regulated a little differently with the FDA. The FDA defines soap as a product that is labeled, sold and represented solely as soap and whose bulk of the nonvolatile matter in the product consists of an alkali salt of salty acids and the product's detergent properties are due to the alkali-fatty acid compounds (FDA, 2009). In this case, soap are regulated by the Consumer Product Safety Commission, no the FDA.

If a product consists of detergents, alkali salts of fatty acids, and is intended not only for cleansing but also to cure, treat, prevent disease or affect the structure or function of the human body than it is regulated as a drug (or as both a drug and cosmetic).

If a product consists of detergents, alkali salts of fatty acids, and is intended only for cleansing the human body and consumers associate with it as soap, then it is regulated as a cosmetic.

Some fragrance products are added to products that are used on the body for treating or preventing disease. Under the law, these types of use are considered drugs, or can be considered as both drugs and cosmetics. Some examples of statements associated with therapeutic uses include, 'easing muscle aches' or 'relieving headaches.'

Massage oils that are intended to lubricate the skin are considered a cosmetic under the FDA rule. But if you claim that the massage oil that you are using will help to relieve muscle aches or reduce a headache, then it could be classified as a drug, or possibly as both a drug and a cosmetic.

How is intended use determined?

There are many ways that one can determine the intended use of a product. They are as follows:

- The ingredients in the product may determine a product's intended use.
- The statement on the label of the product.
- The marketing claims that are made on the product.
- Consumer expectations of the product.

"Essential Oils" and "Aromatherapy"

Even though people use the term, essential oil, to refer to certain oils extracted from plants, the FDA has no regulator definition for the word. Essential oils are commonly used in 'aromatherapy' products and depending on what the product is used for, will depend upon on whether it is classified as a drug, cosmetic or both.

Fragrance Ingredients

In Aromatherapy, we don't consider or use 'fragrance' in our work. We generally use essential oils only. Fragrance is usually a synthetically manufactured substance that does not have any organic connections to it. The FDA does not require approval for fragrances as they are only seen as cosmetic ingredients. Those who manufacture or market cosmetics have a legal responsibility to ensure product safety and proper labeling.

Fragrance and flavor ingredients can be listed as such under U.S. regulations. Both fragrance and flavor formulas are mixtures of natural and synthetic chemical ingredients. The FDA requires a list of ingredients for products sold to the public but it will not force a company to tell its 'trade secrets.' One of the main chemical components in fragrance products is diethyl phthalate (DEP) and is considered safe for human health.

While the FDA has authority to require allergen labeling for food, it does not have the same authority to require allergen labeling for cosmetics. If you have a problem with allergies or sensitive skin, then you may want to choose products that are fragrance free.

What about Setting Standards around the world?

Even though the United States has been lagging behind in setting standards for the quality of essential oils, other countries have moved forward. One such country is France who created the Association Francaise de Normalisation, otherwise known as the Association French Normalization Organization (AFNOR). The organization provides directives and standards for members of the European Union states for companies that wish to exchange good within Europe.

Some of the topics that AFNOR deals with have to do with determining water content, chromatographic profiles, content of phenols, etc.

The United States Pharmacopoeia (USPC) brings standards for medicinal preparations and The National Formulary (NF) set codes for the inactive ingredients that are used in medicine. Today, USPS and NF merged to publish a book called the United States Pharmacopeia-National Formulary (USP-NF), "USP-NF Red Book."

The book provides the FDA with enforceable standards for the quality and strength of health care products. The three volume book contains standards for dosage forms, drug substances, medical devices, medicines and dietary supplements.

Each monograph will include that name of the ingredient, its preparation, packaging, storage, labeling requirements, specifications, tests and procedures for tests, stipulated length, quality and purity.

A   nother organization the deals with setting standards for essential oils is the International Organization for Standardization, (ISO).

The ISO is an independent, non-governmental organization that promotes the development of standardization in the areas of intellectual, scientific, technological, and economic activity. It also provides guidelines for the packaging, conditioning, storage, labeling, sampling and testing of essential oils. ISO is based in Geneva, Switzerland, and it is made up of members from 162 countries around the world. ISO began in 1947 and since then it has published more than 19,500 International Standards covering almost every industry including food safety and healthcare.

The quality of essential oils can be impacted by a variety of environmental factors such as:

Altitude the plant is grown in
Soil Conditions
Amount of Rainfall
Use of Chemicals
Use of Pesticides
Country that the plant is grown in

How do I find quality essential oils?

The Internet lists literally thousands of sources where you can purchase essential oils. But how can you choose which company is legitimate and which oils are top quality? There are a few guidelines and considerations that can help you in locating some good quality oils.

Read the Label. Locate the name of the country where the essential oil comes from. Lavender should come from France, etc. Plants grown in different countries will contain different constituents due to soil, water and air differences. Harvesting and distillation practices may also differ in different countries.

Read the Label. Locate the Latin name of the essential oil that you are looking for to be sure that you are purchasing the right 'species.' Some oils have many different species associated with them and each has a different action.

Smell the oil. The old adage, 'your nose knows' holds true for knowing the difference between good quality essential oils and bad ones.

What's the cost? The real deal will always cost more than the bad ones. If the essential oil is cheap, then it probably is cheap.

Check the producer's statement of purity. Are they claiming that it is 100% pure? Are they guaranteeing the quality?

Does the producer offer information on the how the essential oil was harvested (such as wildcrafting, private farming, etc.) or if it is certified organic?

Did the growers use pesticides or other chemicals while growing the plants to make essential oils?

Are the essential oils processed in a clean facility using good quality standards? Have they been diluted or adulterated in the process? Is it a clean facility or do they pets or rodents running through them?

How are the essential oils handled? Do the people handling the oils wear gloves, masks, etc.?

Are the essential oils packaged properly? Essential oils should be put in dark, glass containers to prevent oxidation.

How are the essential oils stored? Are they properly sealed and then stored in an air-conditioned facility, or are the subject to heat, light or oxygen?

Gas Chromatography and Mass Spectrometry (GC/MS) Testing

GC/MS is the industry standard for identifying different substances in a test sample. This test is used for drug detection, detecting explosives, security, analyzes the atmosphere of other planets, food, aromatic products, and in newborn urine screening tests for more than 100 genetic metabolic disorders. It can detect substances in luggage and on human beings which makes it valuable to forensic experts.

This process of identification began in 1950 when chemists discovered a way to use gas-liquid chromatography to identify substances. But this method proved crude and inefficient. Later, Roland Gohkle and Fred McLafferty developed a new machine that used a mass spectrometer as the detector in gas chromatography. While this worked better than its predecessors, the device was large and fragile and limited to the lab setting.

Twenty years later, an analog-to-digital converter was added to the mass spectrometer which allowed computers to store and interpret the results. By the 20th century, CG-MS machines are now faster and more efficient than ever before.

These machines are used to analyze soil, water and air samples, and in the regulation of food, agriculture and medicines.

This amazing piece of technology can locate each substance in a mixture. How this works is that an operator will dissolve a sample of the object to be analyzed in a liquid and injects that liquid into a stream of gas. The gas will flow through a tube that has been specially coated to catch the compounds as they flow through it. This coating is used to separate each of the substances in the mixture. Each substance will come out of the tube at a different time and when it does, it is ionized and gets an electric charge. An electric magnet is then used to separate the pieces based on their weight. A computer will then measure the pieces and compare them against a computer library of known compounds and makes a list of not only the names of all of the substances in that mixture, but also how much of each substance was in the mixture.

In Aromatherapy, the GC-MS can monitor for organic pollutants in the environment but it may have trouble identifying some pesticides and herbicides as they are too similar to other related compounds. It is however, extensively used for the analysis of such compounds as: esters, fatty acids, alcohols, aldehydes, and terpenes. GC-MS can also be used to detect and measure contaminants from spoilage or adulteration which may be harmful.

When labeling your products, below are some useful resources:

(a) Cosmetic Labeling and Label Claims: An overview to help you get started
(b) Cosmetic Labeling Guide: For step-by-step help that answers many common questions
(c) Cosmetic Labeling Regulations: For links to the full text of the regulations that apply to cosmetic labeling
(d) Some cosmetic labeling requirements are regulated by other federal agencies. For example, the U.S. Federal Trade Commission regulates claims of "Made in USA." Other country of origin labeling is regulated by U.S. Customs and Border Protection (see"Chapter 13-Country of Origin Marking").
(e) You may wish to work with a labeling consultant. FDA, as a government agency, does not provide referrals to private consultants. You may, however, find useful resources under "Trade and Professional Associations of Interest to the Cosmetic Industry" and "Cosmetic Trade Publications."

Harvesting Practices and Procedures

Another thing that affects the quality of essential oils is the harvesting practices and procedures that were followed in producing the essential oil. Some harvesting practices can add different chemical constituents to the essential oil over other practices that could be used to create the same essential oil elsewhere.

Harvesting methods also affect the oil yield and quality. If a plant is harvested at the wrong time of day (or season) the essential oils which are located in the oil glands/veins of the plant, may reduce the amount and quality of the essential oil. An example of this would be the harvesting of cinnamon bark. Normally, the cinnamon bark is harvested during the wet season when the rains have started peeling the bark. Harvesting takes place in the morning before the sun starts to dry out the bark.

Ethics

Ethics is a system of moral principles as it relates to an individual and to a branch of philosophy that deals with the values and conduct of human beings. It is also seen as a rule of conduct in respect to a particular class of humans or groups such as medical ethics or business ethics. Ethics can also deal with actions that are seen as being either 'right' or 'wrong' and 'good' or 'bad.'

Many regulating and professional organizations will have a 'code of ethics' to which its membership must adhere to. This code of ethics is a set of guiding moral principles that is set out to govern the individual's course of action. A failure to do so would result in the organization to take action against the individual by either reprimand, loss of membership and even loss of licensure.

The code of ethics is important to any profession as it speaks to the integrity of both the group and the individual. Most of these codes include verbiage on honesty, anti-discriminatory procedures, confidentiality, professional boundaries, quality of care, scope of practice, informed consent, sexual contact, standards of practice and ethical decision making.

Ethical Decision Making

When a client comes to you for help, they are putting themselves in a place of trust. You must respect trust relationship and do your best in making decisions concerning the health of your client. Not only must you be respectful of this imbalance of power, but you must also be ethical. The client has put their trust in you and your knowledge to help them with an issue.

You must make sure that the decision that you make for them (such as a course of treatment), is in their best interest and will not injure or harm them.

Referrals

If you find that you client could benefit from a modality, or course of treatment, that is outside of your scope of practice or abilities, then you should give them a referral. This is not only the professional thing to do; it is the ethical thing to do.

The only problem with referring a client to another profession is if you get a kick-back from that professional. If you do receive something in exchange for the referral, then you run the risk of breaking the law in the United States.

Please be aware that if you give your client the name of another therapist, then you must also give them at least two other names of therapists in the same field. This is the law. The law that I am mentioning here is called the Stark and Anti-Kickback law that regulates the relationship between physicians and other healthcare providers.

The purpose of the law was to prevent physicians (and other healthcare providers) from referring a patient for certain services and then receiving a reimbursement for the referral. The act was meant to stop unnecessary testing. Violation of this law may result in a monetary penalty of up to $15,000 per violation and $100,000 per arrangements or overall scheme.

The Anti-Kickback Statute is a criminal statute that prohibits the willful solicitation or acceptance of any type of remuneration to induce referrals for health services. Remuneration includes savings on rental space (or free rent), percentage of client payments, free services, free education, or any other perks. Violations of this statute may result in a monetary penalty of up to $50,000 per violation.

Prescription vs. Referral Form

A prescription is a written order from a physician or nurse practitioner authorizing a specific treatment. These orders are written on the physicians prescription pad and should include date, client's name, diagnosis and code, treatment order, frequency of treatments, duration of treatments and referring health care provider's name, signature and contact information.

Prescriptions are usually given for medication, therapy, or therapeutic devices. If a therapist accepts a prescription for therapy, then you provide ONLY what is listed on the prescription and be sure to document your service for the referring healthcare professional. The client would then return to the referring health care provider for their follow-up and evaluation. Therapist should retain the original prescription and add it to the client's file.

You can make copies for the client or referring physician, or for the insurance company, but you should always retain the original copy for yourself.

A referral form is generally produced by the healthcare provider (which can be you), and is given to and filled out by, the health care provider authorizing a specific treatment. These forms can contain the information listed above (except for the diagnosing part if you are not qualified to diagnose a condition).

Code of Ethics
The following is the Code of Ethics from the National Association of Holistic Aromatherapy (NAHA).

1.1 Demonstrate commitment to provide the highest quality aromatherapy service to those who seek their professional service

1.2 Conduct myself in a professional and ethical manner in relation to my clients, fellow aromatherapists & colleagues and the general public so as to comply with the highest standards of moral behavior & integrity and to uphold the dignity and status of my profession under all circumstances.

1.3 Share professional knowledge, research, and experiences with fellow aromatherapists/colleagues to support the advancement of aromatherapy.

1.4 Treat clients in accordance with holistic principles (Recommend treatment based upon the specific needs of the client.) and render professional services for no other purposes than the total well-being of my clients.

1.5 Educate clients in the quality and availability of true aromatherapy products and services.

1.6 Refrain from engaging in any sexual conduct or sexual activities involving clients.

1.7 Recognize that my primary obligation is always to the client and agree to practice Aromatherapy to the best of my ability for my client's benefit. Client's comfort, welfare and health must always have priority.

1.8 Provide clients with informed consent/disclosure statement and information that includes training, certification, scope of practice,
payment structure, benefits, limitations and expectations of both the practitioner and client.

1.9 Endeavor to serve the best interests of my clients at all times by providing the highest quality of service and I shall undertake continuing education and improve upon my Aromatherapy skills and professional standards whenever possible.

1.10 Provide services within the scope and the limits of my training. I will not employ techniques for which I have not had adequate training and shall represent my education, training, qualifications and abilities honestly. I shall acknowledge the limitations of my skills and when necessary, refer clients to the appropriate qualified professionals.

1.11 Not diagnose, prescribe or provide any service, which requires a license to practice unless specifically licensed to do.

1.12 Maintain client confidentiality and not divulge the findings I acquire during consultation, or in the course of professional recommendations, without my clients consent except when required by law.

1.13 Support other Consultants at all time and shall never criticize, condemn or otherwise denigrate other Consultants in the presence of a client or other lay persons.

1.14 Respect the rights of other healthcare professionals and aromatherapists and will cooperate with all health care professionals in a friendly and professional manner.

1.15 Where another Consultant refers a client to me, I shall return such clients to the original Consultant when the specified recommendation is completed. I will not denigrate another Consultant's recommendations.

1.16 Not make false claims regarding the potential benefits of Aromatherapy and shall actively participate in educating the public regarding the actual benefits of True Aromatherapy.

1.17 Not give guarantees regarding the results of any recommendations, nor exploit a client for financial gain through inferences or misrepresentation of any sort.

1.18 Practice honesty in advertising, promote my services ethically and in good taste, and practice and or advertise only those skills for which I have received adequate training or certification.

1.19 Maintain my premises in a hygienic condition, and ensure that my premises offer my Clients sufficient privacy.

1.20 Maintain complete records of each Client, including specific details of my recommendations.

1.21 Refrain from the use of any mind-altering drugs, alcohol, or intoxicants prior to or during a professional Aromatherapy consultation or while representing the National Association for Holistic Aromatherapy.

1.22 Dress in a professional manner, proper dress being defined as the attire suitable and consistent with accepted professional practice.

1.23 Represent a united front to the public and refrain from criticism of colleagues either in writing or verbally before clients or the public.

1.24 Shall, upon being found to have transgressed any of the By-laws of the National Association for Holistic Aromatherapy and/or this Code of Ethics voluntarily surrender and return my membership certificate to the Association.

Chapter Fourteen
Some Recipes

Below is a quick chart of some of the more popular essential oils to use with your canine friend:

Quick Chart for Selecting Oils for your Canine

Essential Oil	Identifying Name	Use to:
Atlas Cedarwood	Cedrus atlantica	Insect Repellent including moths from storage Grounds and stabilizes the nervous system Use in shampoo (>1% dilution) to repels fleas and ticks, mosquitoes, etc. May stop hair loss that is due to stress Treats dry skin conditions Relieves rheumatic and arthritic pain
Frankincense	Boswelia fereana	Relieves Distress, comforts, calms, PTS, Relieve Insecurity, anxiety, grief and loss
German Chamomile	Matricaria recutita	Anti-inflammatory, Antispasmodic. Anti-fungal, Anti-septic, Insect Repellent, Stimulates production of red blood cells, Relieves aches and pains. Analgesic,

		Treats inflamed and irritated skin conditions, boils, rashes, dermatisic, eczema and psoriasis Treats burns, cuts, and calms/soothes emotions
Lavender	Lavandula angustifolia	Anti-bacterial, Anti-fungal, heal wounds, Prevent blistering, balance moods, depression, Stress, fear, and irritability
Lemongrass	Cymbopogon citratus	Anti-fungal, astringent, Insect Repellent, Anti-inflammatory, Sedative (CNS) Regulates oily skin, Relieves muscle spasms, Promotes regeneration/healing of soft tissue,
Neroli	Citrus aurantium	Relieves stress and anxiety, uplifts emotions, Helpful for depression and shock
Niaouli	Melaleuca quinquenervia virdiflora	Anti-fungal, Antiseptic, Antibacterial, Anti-viral, Use to treat thrust or horse hoof fungal infection,
Patchouli	Pogostemon cablin	Anti-fungal, Antiseptic, Insect Repellent Treats fleas and ticks, soothes skin bites, Tones and strengthens skin cell tissue Regulates oily and combination skin issues Controls skin infections and outbreaks
Rose Geranium	Pelargonium roseum	Insect Repellent, Balancing, Calming, Uplifting, Treats hormonal imbalance and

		CNS, Treats fleas and ticks
Sweet Marjoram	Origanum marjorana	Anti-spasmodic, Analgesic, Treats muscles spasms, strains and sprains Treats joint stiffness and pain
Thyme	Thymus vulgaris CT. linalool	Anti-microbial, Anti-bacterial, Immune Stimulant (Do NOT use on cats, birds or near fish tanks)

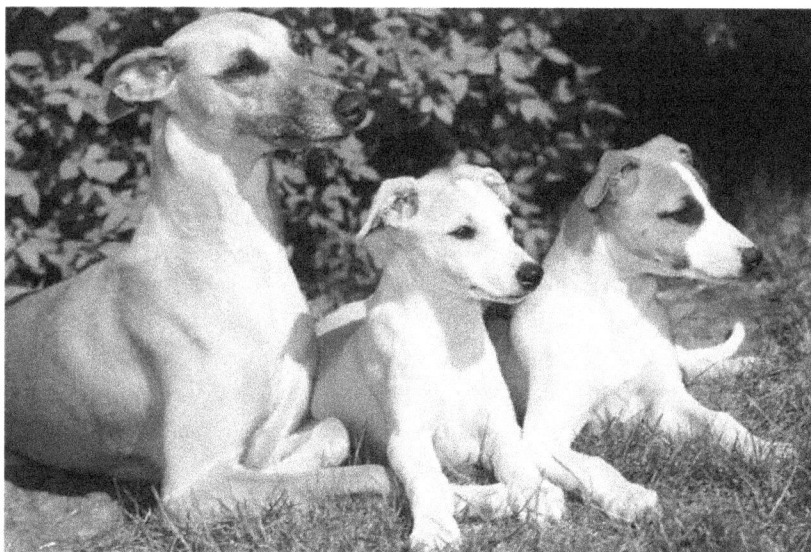

1. Pet Spray for Fleas

Ingredients:
   8 ounces of distilled water or boiled tap water
   20 drops of Lavender essential oil
   20 drops of Orange essential oil
   15 drops of Tea Tree essential oil
   5 drops of Lemongrass essential oil
   1 eight ounce spray bottle

To Do:

To make this soothing spray, you will need to use some distilled water or just boil some tap water.

Use an eight ounce spray bottle and fill it with the water leaving about ½ inch from the top empty.

Shake the bottle thoroughly before each spray application.

Use this spray after you have bathed your animal. It is a good idea to spray your pet outdoors, away from your house, because the fleas will jump off the animal once the spray is on them. Be sure to work the spray into your animal's coat a bit. None of the essential oils listed above are in enough concentration to actually kill fleas, but they will make the flea's stay on your pet a very uncomfortable one until they decide to leave.

The spray will also help to ease and soothe minor skin irritations and help to heal minor scrapes, cuts and bites.

You can also use this spray as a preventative to keep fleas from ever attacking your pet in the first place. If needed, this spray can also be used as a deodorizer for your pet.

2. Pest Powder

Ingredients:
    4 ounces of arrowroot
    20 drops of Pennyroyal essential oil
    20 drops of Lemongrass essential oil
    15 drops of Tea Tree essential oil
    10 drops of Citronella essential oil
    1 shaker container

To Do:

To make this Pest Powder, you will need a large mixing bowl and a mixing utensil, or a blender.

Place the arrowroot powder into the mixing bowl or blender and add all of the essential oils as listed above. Blend well.

When finished, pour blend into a shaker container and be sure to date and label it.

Sprinkle this blend on your pet, and their bedding or favorite napping place, to repel fleas, ticks and other bothersome pests.

Try a test patch on a piece of your carpet before you sprinkle this blend on your entire carpeted area. Essential oils can stain some furniture and carpeting, so be safe-not sorry.

If you cannot find arrowroot, you can substitute this powder with regular baking soda. The baking soda is much cheaper and more easily available in most locations.

3. Dental Care Paste

Ingredients:
>**2 tablespoons of regular baking soda**
>**2 drops of water**
>**1 drop of Anise essential oil**
>**1 drop of Clove essential oil**
>**1 piece of cotton**

To Do:

Mix all of the above ingredients (except the piece of cotton) together in a jar or small container.

Use a piece of cotton, or wool, instead of a toothbrush to brush your pet's teeth. Toothbrushes can sometimes harm your pet's gums.
Simply dampen the cloth and dip it into your baking soda mixture. Now, gently pass the cloth over as many teeth as possible while trying to avoid scrubbing too hard.

The essential oils in this past will also work as disinfectants and deodorizers for the pet. This blend is partially numbing for the relief of minor toothaches.

If your pet is already suffering from a dental problem then this blend is not going to help. Please take your pet to the veterinarian for proper treatment.

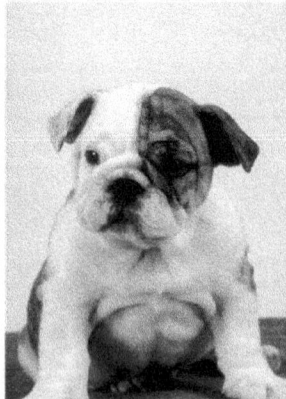

4. For Cracked and Scaly Skin

Ingredients:
3-5 drops of Sandalwood essential oil
2 ounces of Sweet Almond carrier oil
1 glass container

To Do:
Combine all ingredients together into the glass container.
Shake well before each use.
Gentle rub the blend into the pet's skin to help moisturize it.
You can use this blend at the first sight of skin problems and irritations.
Apply the blend directly to your pet's skin.

If you pet really dislikes the smell of the essential oil, then you can dilute this blend by adding more Sweet Almond carrier oil. Each pet is different and each one has their own tolerance level. Do a patch test first and see how your pet reacts to it before applying the blend to their whole body.

Please realize that your pet can also change their mind from day to day depending on their mood. You may have to readjust the blend several times over the next few days to keep your pet happy.

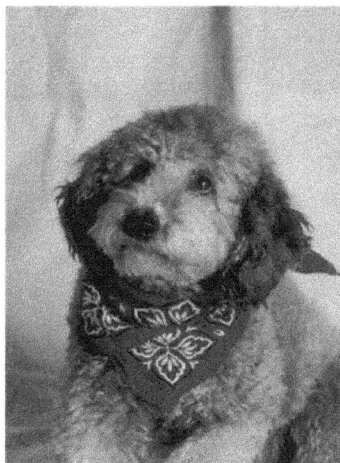

5. A Happy Cat Pest Collar

Ingredients:
- ½ teaspoon of alcohol
- 1 drop of Cedarwood essential oil
- 1 drop of Lavender essential oil
- 1 drop of Citronella essential oil
- 1 drop of Thyme essential oil
- 1 drop of Garlic oil
- 1 teaspoon of vegetable oil

To Do:

Mix all of the ingredients together and dip your pet's collar into the mixture until it is completely absorbed. Be sure that the collar is dry before placing it around your cat's neck.

If your cat appears in discomfort due to the essential oils, please discard the collar and skip using essential oils on your pet.

Collar should be effective up to 1 month.

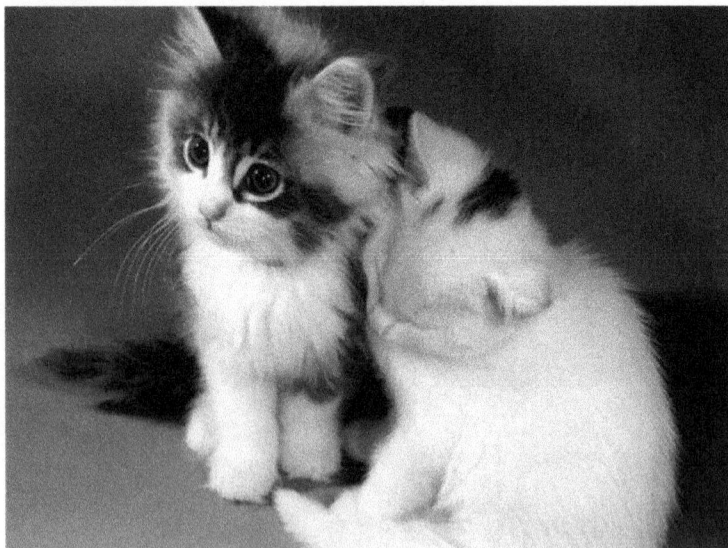

6. Pet Bath Time

Ingredients
2 gallons of bath water
8 drops of essential oil

To Do:
Add your choice of 8 drops of essential oil to every 2 gallons of water that you use for your pet's bath.

You can pick from the following essential oils for your pet's enjoyment.

Eucalyptus
Lavender
Cedarwood
Peppermint

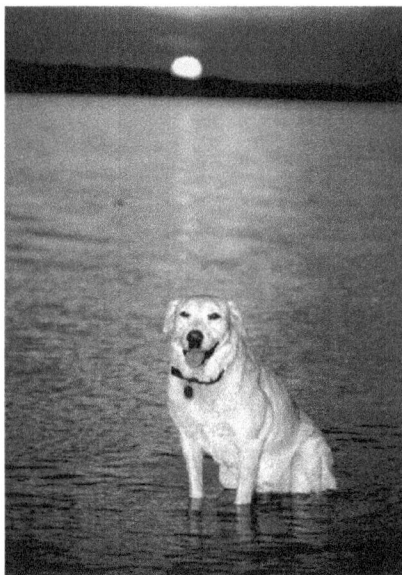

7. Bad Breath

Ingredients:
   1 teaspoon of vegetable oil
   1 drop of essential oil (choose from clove, lavender or myrrh)

If bad breath is caused by dental problems, I would use the clove which has a numbing effect.

If bad breath is caused by mouth sores, I would use lavender or myrrh If bad breath is caused by stomach problems, I would use myrrh

If bad breath is caused by something the dog just chewed on, I would use the lavender.

To Do:
   Add 1 drop of the essential oil that you chose from above to the 1 teaspoon of vegetable oil and use a pet toothbrush, or soft cloth, to apply the mixture to your pet's teeth.

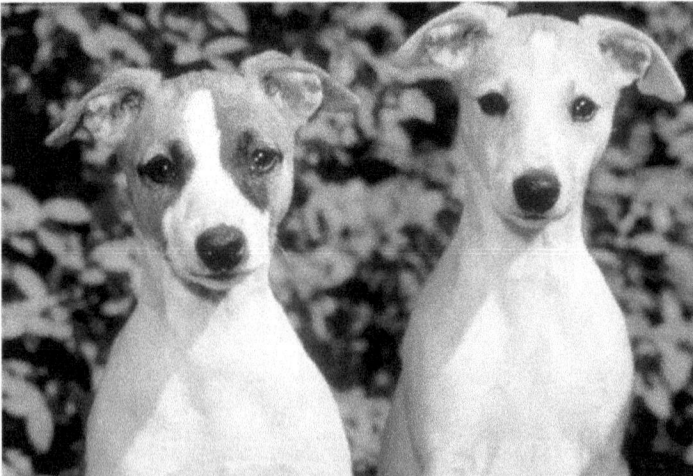

8. Ear Problems

Ingredients:
> **1 drop of Helichrysum essential oil**
> **1 drop of lavender essential oil**
> **1 drop of roman chamomile essential oil**
> **1 teaspoon of olive oil**

To Do:
You will first warm the olive oil. My mother always did this by placing the olive oil in a teaspoon and she would run a candle under the spoon until the oil was warm. Please be very careful here and don't make the oil too warm or hot as it can damage your poor pet's ear.

Once you have the oil slightly warmed, add the three essential oils as listed above and blend well.

Drop the blend into your pet's affected ear and gently massage the area around the ear.

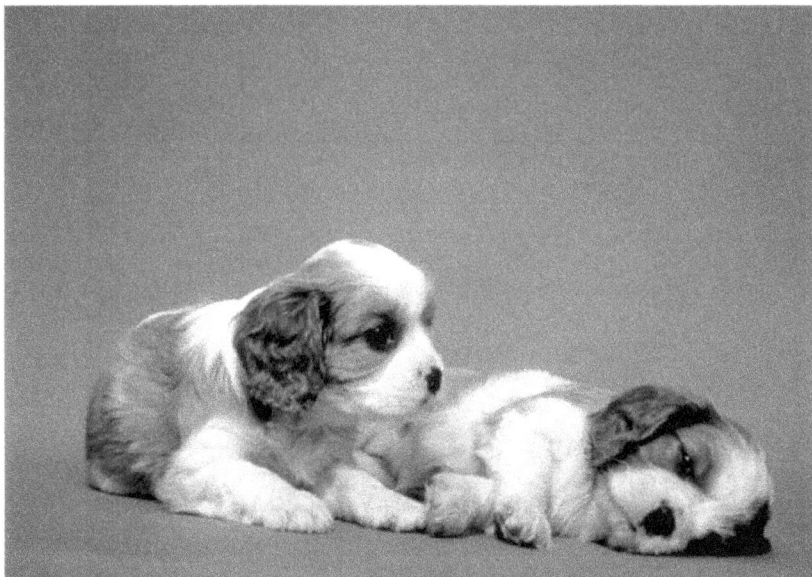

9.   Anxiousness and Hyperactivity Spray

Ingredients:
>1 drop of Clary Sage essential oil
>1 drop of Lavender essential oil
>1 drop of Ylang Ylang essential oil
>4 ounces of distilled water

To Do:
>Place the essential oils and water in a spray bottle and shake well. Spray your pet's bed or sleeping area.

Just like people and children, pets too experience emotions of fear, anxiety and uncertainty. Pets also experience anger and stress which causes many of them to act nervous. Ever see a dog shiver or shake from fright?

This spray will help to calm nerves, alleviate anxiety and to relax the mind. This spray will be good for the pet owner too.

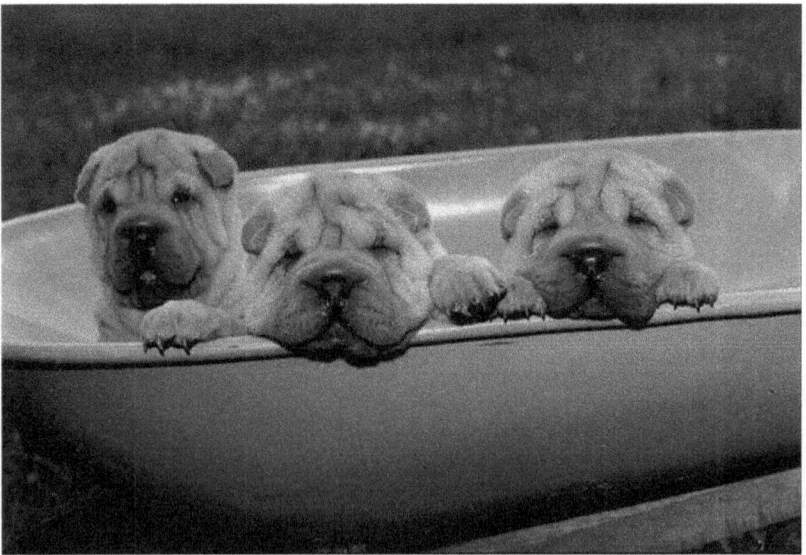

10. Arthritis

Ingredients:
    1 drop of Ginger essential oil
    1 drop of Lavender essential oil
    2 drops of Rosemary essential oil
    1 tablespoon of vegetable oil

To Do:
    Blend together all of the above ingredients into a glass container.

    Put some of the blend on your fingertips and thumb and rub them together until you can feel nice warmth coming from your fingertips.

    Now begin to gently massage your pet in slow movements starting from bottom of the dogs legs up to the back and then gently massage your pet's back from the bottom of the vertebrae up to the head.

    Reapply blend to your fingertips as needed. Remember, if you have a large dog, you will want to double the recipe above.

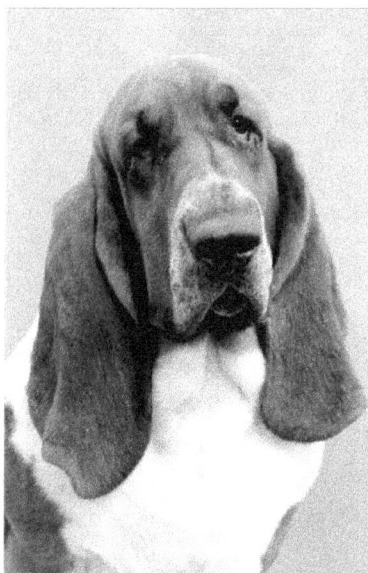

11. Ear Wax

Ingredients
    3 drops of Lavender essential oil
    1 teaspoon of Witch Hazel

To Do:
    Mix the essential oil in the Witch Hazel.
    Use a dropper to in take the mixture and insert it into the pet's ear.
    Massage the ear on the outside for one minute.

Repeat this process daily until the wax is softened enough to be removed safely with a cotton wool.

Do not perform this exercise if the pet finds this painful, take your pet to your veterinarian immediately.

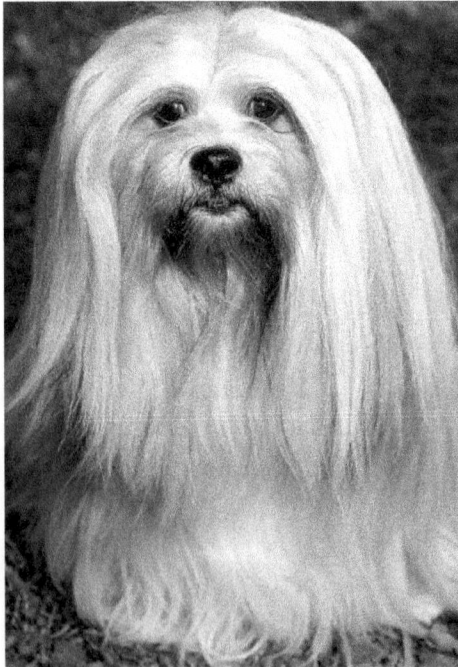

12. First-Aid for Cuts

Ingredients:
6 drops of Lavender essential oil
½ gallon of water

To Do:
Combine the essentials oils to the water.

Use the water solution to cleanse any of your pet's wounds and abrasions.

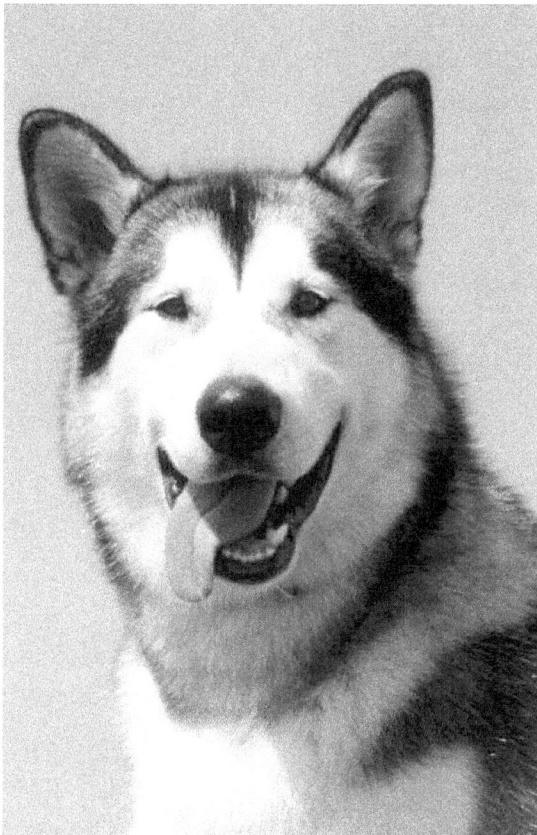

13. Bronchitis

Ingredients:
    2 drops of Eucalyptus essential oil
    6 teaspoons of water

NOTE: If you have a large dog, you can double and even triple this recipe as follows:

    4 drops of essential oil to 12 teaspoons of water
    6 drops of essential oil to 18 teaspoons of water

To Do:
    Warm the water slightly
    Combine the essential oils and water.
    Place a cloth into the mixture until it is soaked. Squeeze out the excess water.
    Place the damp cloth on your pet's chest for 1 minute.
    Remove the cloth and place a dry blanket over your pet to keep the area warm.
    If this appears to help your pet, you can reapply again in 8 hours.

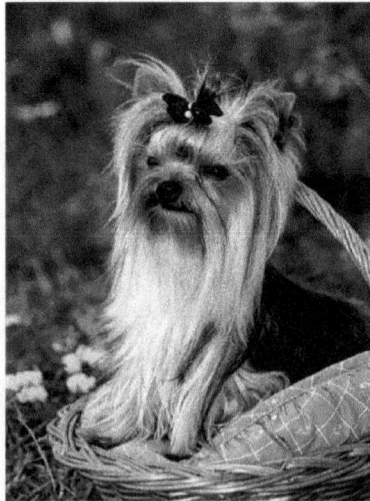

14. For a Shinier Coat

Ingredients:
5 drops of Carrot essential oil
5 drops of Evening Primrose essential oil
1 drop of Rosemary essential oil
1 tablespoon of Wheatgerm oil
1 tablespoon of Olive Oil

To Do:
Combine all of the above ingredients together and massage into your pet's coat.

Allow the mixture to soak into the coat for at least 3-5 minutes. Now, shampoo as regular.

Can be used as a coat conditioner once a week.

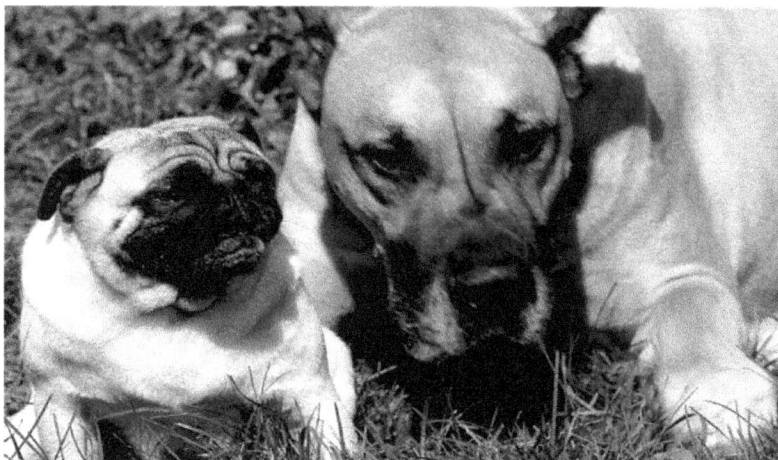

15. For Itching Relief

Ingredients:
    5 drops of Geranium essential oil
    4 drops of Lavender essential oil
    3 drops of Roman Chamomile oil
    1 ounce of Olive Oil

To Do:
    Mix above ingredients together and gently apply the blend to the areas of your pet most affected.
    You can use a cotton ball to apply the mixture, your fingertips or a cloth soaked in the mixture.
    Reapply as needed. Your pet should have relief by the end of the day if you can reapply the blend at least three times throughout the day.

NOTE: If you prefer not to use the Olive Oil, you can use other carrier oils such as jojoba. I like to use olive oil where healing is needed.

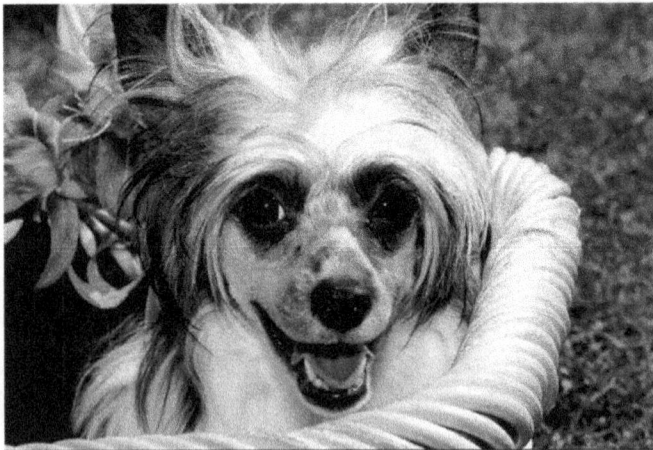

16. Rheumatism Relief

Ingredients:
> 4 drops of Birch essential oil
> 4 drops of Juniper essential oil
> 3 drops of Rosemary essential oil
> 1 ounce of carrier oils (choose between calendula, jojoba or
> vegetable)

To Do:
Combine all of the above ingredients together and gently massage your pet with the blend in the morning and again at night before retiring.

You can also through your pet's blanket into the dryer for 5 minutes to slightly warm it.

Most pets who suffer from rheumatism and arthritis love to find a hot spot on the floor to lie on.

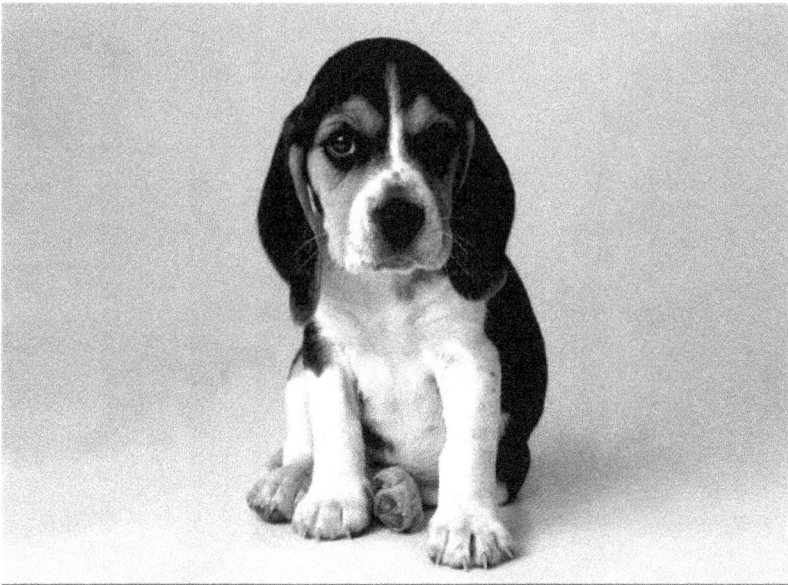

17. Energy Booster

Ingredients:
>   **4 drops of Lavender essential oil**
>   **3 drops of Rosemary essential oil**
>   **1 drop of Peppermint essential oil**
>   **1 ounce of carrier oil (your choice)**

To Do:

Mix all of the above ingredients together and place some of the blend on a cotton ball and 'dab' the mixture down your pet's spine.

Please note, if your pet does NOT like this blend, try diluting it with more carrier oil. Peppermint tends to be VERY strong so dilute it until you can barely smell it anymore.

Do NOT use this blend in the evening as it will disrupt your pet's sleep.

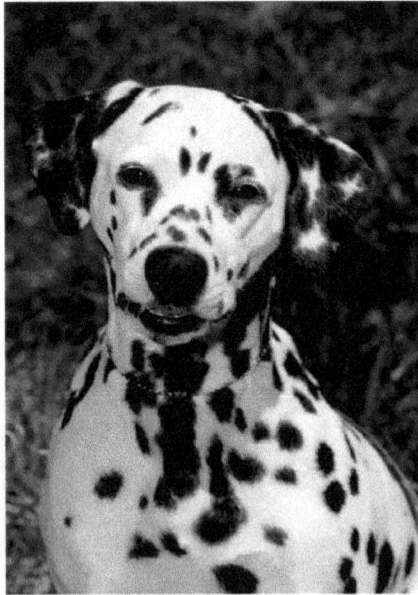

18. For Pet Odor

Ingredients:
    6 drops of Lavender essential oil
    6 drops of Geranium essential oil
    3 drops of Lemon essential oil
    1 drop of Pine essential oil
    1 ounce spray bottle filled with distilled water

To Do:
    Combine all of the above ingredients together and shake well. Spray the blend directly on your dog.
    Avoid spraying directly on your pets' eyes, nose or mouth.

You can spray your pet's sleeping area. Do NOT soak the area.
    Be warned that certain oils will stain carpet and furniture.

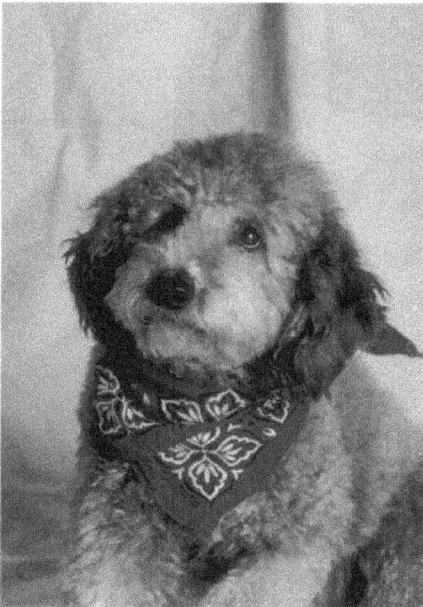

19. For Stress

Ingredients
- **4 drops of Lavender essential oil**
- **2 drops of Marjoram essential oil**
- **1 drop of Neroli essential oil**
- **1 ounce of carrier oil (choose from Sweet Almond, jojoba or calendula)**

To Do:

Combine all the above ingredients together and apply to your pet using a cloth or your fingertips.

Use slow, gently and comforting strokes and speak in a slow, loving and comforting voice.

Repeat as needed

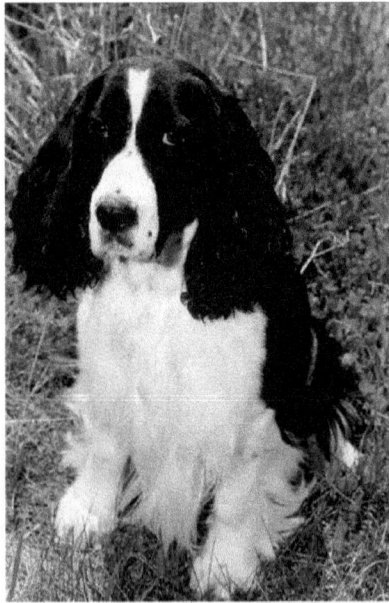

20. For Lonliness

Ingredients:
>**4 drops of Marjoram essential oil**
>**3 drops of Cypress essential oil**
>**2 drops of Rose Otto essential oil**
>**1 ounce of carrier oil (choose from jojoba, Sweet Almond or Calendula)**

To Do:

Combine all of the ingredients above together and slowly and gently rub the blend into the pet.

Be sure to keep your strokes gentle and loving and reassure your pet all the way.

Use this blend when there has been a death in the family, a traumatic experience, or a move to a new location.

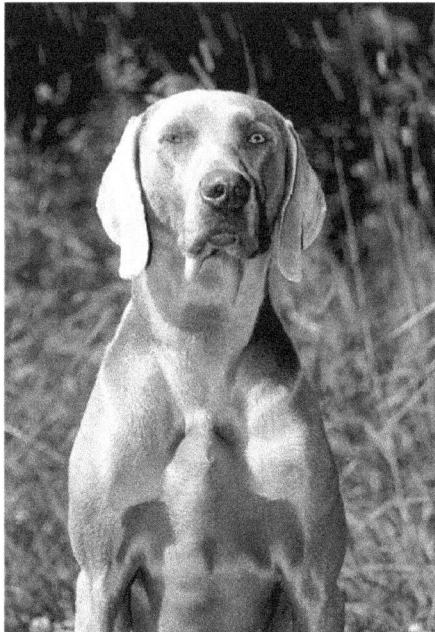

21. Anxiousness

Ingredients:
- **4 drops of Lavender essential oil**
- **2 drops of Petitgrain essential oil**
- **1 drop of Roman Chamomile essential oil**
- **1 drop of Rose Otto essential oil**
- **1 ounce of carrier oil (choose from vegetable, jojoba or Sweet Almond)**

To Do:

Combine all of the ingredients above and massage your pet gently with the blend.

Remember that pets react to your own emotions. If you are anxious, they will be anxious too. They can sense that something is not right and then they 'act' out your frustrations, fears and nervousness.

The best thing you can do for a nervous pet is to calm yourself down. Try sitting on a nice blanket or on the couch or chair, with the television off and just stroke and speak to your pet in a slow and calm manner. A super great way to calm both of you down at the same time!

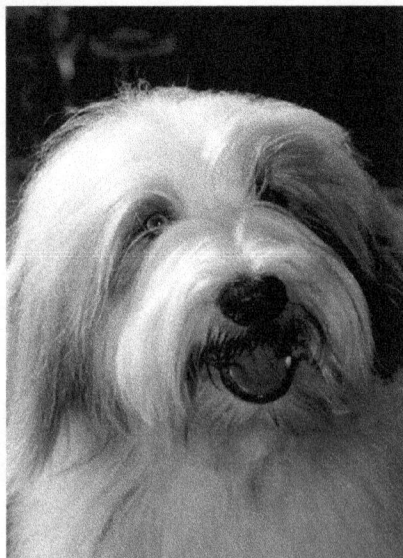

Natural Health Care Tips

Abscesses- Put 1 drop of lavender or helichrysum essential oil directly on the abscess. When pus is discharged, put 1 drop of lavender essential oil on the area and then clean the area with a salt and water mixture.

Cuts and Bites- Bathe the entire area that is affected with a solution of salt and water to which you have added 2 drops of thyme essential oil. After you have washed the area with the mixture, apply 1 drop of lavender essential oil directly to the affected area.

Cysts- Apply 1 drops of lavender essential oil, or 1 drop of tea tree oil, directly to the cyst. Reapply as needed.

Anal Swelling- Blend together 5 drops of roman chamomile essential oil and 5 drops of tea tree essential oil into 1 teaspoon of vegetable oil. Apply to the affected area using

Added Hints:

- Bathe your pet once with plain mild shampoo and cold water first before using the orange shampoo.
- Make the experience of powdering and spraying as enjoyable as you can for your pet.
- Be sure to label and date all of your products so that you know what they are and can dispose of them when they have expired. A shelf life for most essential oils is 1 month.
- Do not use citrus oils on pets as they may irritate their skin
- Add 5 drops of lavender and Cedarwood essential oils to pet pillows and mattresses.

Glossary of Terms

Analgesic: Pain relieving. Agent or remedy that helps to deaden pain.
Antibacterial: Destroys bacteria
Antifungal: Destroys fungus and mold
Anti-inflammatory (Antiphlogistic): Reduces inflammation
Antispasmodic: Relieves spasms and cramping
Antiviral: Destroys viruses
Aphrodisiac: Promotes sexual desire
Carminative: Expulsion of gas from the intestines
Cholagogue: Elimination of bile from the gall bladder, bile ducts
Cicatrizant: Promotes healing by scar formation at the location of a healing wound
Decongestant: Expels excess fluid in sinuses, tissues and membranes
Deodorant: Eliminates body odors
Diaphoretic: Increases perspiration or sweat
Emmenahogue: Promotes menstruation
Expectorant: Promotes expulsion of mucus
Febrifuge: Fever reducing
Hepatic: Relating to the liver. Relaxes the liver and tones and aids its function.
Nervine: Supports and strengthens the nervous system and nerves
Purgative: Stimulates the movement of the bowels
Relaxant: Calms or relaxes nerves, organ, body and/or mind
Rubefacient: Causes redness of the skin
Stimulant: Increases circulation, movements of body, mind or spirit
Stomachic: Stomach stimulant or tonic, improves appetite
Vulnerary: Heals Wounds and sores by external application

About the Author

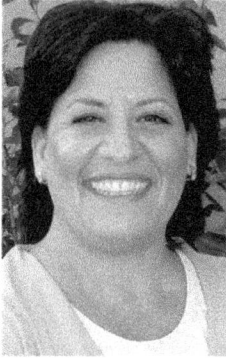

Francine Milford, BS, LMT, CTN

Francine Milford, BS, LMT, CTN, is a state and nationally licensed massage therapist and personal trainer who resides in Venice, Florida where she is the owner of the Reiki Center of Venice. At the Center, Francine teaches more than 70 different modalities of Alternative Therapies which include Bach Flower, Aromatherapy, Herbology, Homeopathy, Chakra Energy Work and Reiki Natural System of Healing.

Francine is a continuing education provider for the National Certifying Board of Therapeutic Massage and Bodywork (NCBTMB) and BOC, the National Athletic Trainers Association, as well as, for the State of Florida Massage Therapy Board.

The Reiki Center of Venice offers two levels of Aromatherapy Correspondence Courses a total 250 hour program of professional study. Level One is 50 hours in length and Level Two is 200 hours of training.

To learn more about this wonderful course which is easy to understand and with directions that is easy to follow, order yours today. You can view what is included in your purchase on the website before you make your decision. This course is the best priced course on the market today. You won't be sorry you did. Visit www.AromaCareBooks.com.

References

Badcock, Laura (2008, Dec. 18). *Absorption & elimination of essential oils.* Web. Retrieved from http://www.essentialwholesale.com/library/absorption-elimination-of-essential-oils.

Battaglia, S. (2003). *The complete guide to aromatherapy.* 2nd ed. The Perfect Potion. Pty Ltd.Buckle, J. (2003). *Clinical aromatherapy: Essential oils in practice, 2nd Ed.* Edinburgh: Churchill Livingstone.

Cooksley, Valerie Gennari. (1996). *Aromatherapy: a lifetime guide to healing with essential oils.* Prentice Hall.
Halcón, Linda and Maher, Kater. (2013, July 16). *How do I determine the quality of essential oils.* The University of Minnesota. Web. Retrieved from http://www.takingcharge.csh.umn.edu/explore-healing-practices/aromatherapy/how-do-i-determine-quality-essential-oils.

Hochell, Jennifer. (2006). *Introduction to Aromatherapy.* Home Study Course and Certification.

Hochell, Jennifer. (2006). *Advanced Aromatherapy.* Home Study Course and Certification.

Jones L. (1998) "Establishing standards for essential oils and analytical standards" *Proceedings of NAHA The World of Aromatherapy II International Conference and Trade Show* St. Louis, Missouri, Sept 25-28, 1998, p146-163.

Lawless, Julia. (1997). *The complete illustrated guide to aromatherapy, a practical approach to the use of essential oils for health and well-being.* Element Books Limited.

Lawless, Julia. (1995). *The illustrated encyclopedia of essential oils, the complete guide to the use of oils in aromatherapy and herbalism.* Element Books Limited.

Lyth, Geoff. 2002. *Sources and origins of our essential oils.* Quinessence Aromatherapy. Retrieved from http://www.quinessence.com/essential_oil_origins.htm.
Margaret, Ingrid. (2006). *Aromatherapy for massage practitioners.* Lippincott Williams & Wilkins.

Price, S. & Price, L. (2007). Aromatherapy for health professionals, 3rd Ed. Philadelphia: Churchill Livingstone Elsevier.

Salvo, Susan. (2007). *Massage therapy principles and practice.* 3rd Edition. Saunders Elsevier.

Salvo, Susan. (2007). *Massage therapy principles and practice.* 3rd Edition. Saunders Elsevier.

Shannon, J.C. (2012, August 7). *Curbing cravings and assaulting addictions with essential oils.* Web. Retrieved from http://essentialhealth.com/2012/08/curbing-cravings-and-assaulting-addictions-with-essential-oils.

Thibodeau and Patton. (2008). *Structure and function of the body.* 13th ed. Mosby, Inc.Tisserand, R. & Balacs, T. (1995). *Essential oil safety: A guide for health professionals.* Edinburgh: Churchill Livingstone.

U.S. Food and Drug Administration (FDA). (2009). Fragrances in Cosmetics. Web. Retrieved from http://www.fda.gov/Cosmetics/ProductsIngredients.

Williams, D.G. (1997). *The chemistry of essential oils: an introduction for aromatherapists, beauticians, retailers and students.* England: Micelle Press.

Worwood, Valerie Ann. (1991). *The complete book of essential oils & aromatherapy.* New World Library.

Websites:

Visit www.AromaCareBooks.com for sfree information, tips and blends.

Visit www.ReikiCenterofVenice.com for upcoming classes and health articles.

Visit www.Naha.org for information on Aromatherapy

www.ingramcontent.com/pod-product-compliance
Lightning Source LLC
Chambersburg PA
CBHW030011290326
41934CB00005B/296